# Aids to Reproductive Biology

# Aids to Reproductive Biology For MRCOG Part I

**Gordon M. Stirrat**

MA MD FRCOG

Professor of Obstetrics and Gynaecology
Bristol Maternity Hospital, Bristol

*Foreword by*

**A. C. Turnbull**

MA MD FRCOG

Nuffield Professor of Obstetrics and Gynaecology
John Radcliffe Hospital, Oxford

CHURCHILL LIVINGSTONE
EDINBURGH LONDON MELBOURNE AND NEW YORK 1983

CHURCHILL LIVINGSTONE
Medical Division of Longman Group Limited

Distributed in the United States of America by
Churchill Livingstone Inc., 19 West 44 Street, New
York, N.Y. 10036, and by associated companies,
branches and representatives throughout the
world.

First published 1983

ISBN 0 443 02233 X

British Library Cataloguing in Publication Data
Stirrat, Gordon M.
   Aids to reproductive biology.
   1. Human reproduction
   I. Title
   612′.6        QP251

Library of Congress Cataloging in Publication Data
Stirrat, Gordon M.
   Aids to reproductive biology.

   Includes bibliographical references and index.
   1. Human reproduction. I. Title. [DNLM:
1. Obstetrics — Outlines. 2. Reproduction — Outlines. 3. Pregnancy —
Outlines. WQ 18 S861a]
QP251.S848      612.6        82–4249
                           AACR2

Printed in Singapore by
Huntsmen Offset Printing Pte Ltd.

# Foreword

Knowledge has been expanding rapidly in the field of reproductive biology, particularly in recent years, and it is therefore especially helpful at this time to have the main aspects brought together in such a compact, authoritative *Aids to Reproductive Biology*. Professor Gordon Stirrat is to be congratulated on the production of a book which provides so much information so succinctly; the writing is crisp, unequivocal and clearly understandable. The emphasis throughout is on human reproduction. The text is divided into sections, the largest of which is reproductive biology, while the other sections include developmental biology, maternal accommodation to pregnancy, parturition, the puerperium, and general clinical physiology.

*Aids to Reproductive Biology* provides a solid basis of understanding of the field and will be most valuable for both undergraduates and postgraduates. Of course, reproductive biology is an essential part of the scientific basis of clinical obstetrics and gynaecology. This book will therefore be of particular value for postgraduates working for a higher qualification in that specialty because it deals with most of the basic reproductive science required for the first part of the examination for MRCOG. Naturally, a book as condensed as this cannot be complete or comprehensive, and it should be regarded as a guide rather than as a specific text; however, each section lists suggestions for further reading.

*Aids to Reproductive Biology* describes and elucidates the main aspects of a field of great and increasing importance. I am sure it will prove to be the constant companion of all who wish to learn more about this fascinating science.

A.C.T.

# Preface

This book aims to provide a synoptic guide to the essentials of reproductive biology. It is written primarily but not solely with candidates for the MRCOG (Part 1) examination in mind.

It cannot, by its very nature, be totally comprehensive and readers are encouraged to supplement their knowledge from among the books in the suggested further reading lists which follow every section and to make notes in the blank sheets provided.

More clinical pharmacology and pathology than is contained here needs to be covered for the MRCOG Part I, but the author craves the indulgence of the reader in that they have been placed within the appropriate clinical context in *Aids to Obstetrics and Gynaecology** General pathology is covered well by another title in this series — *Aids to Pathology* by Dr Michael Dixon.

The work of a multitude of eminent authors has contributed to the body of knowledge summarised in this book and its clinical counterpart and my debt to them is gratefully acknowledged.

I would particularly like to thank the following authors and publishers for permission to reproduce the material listed below: Mitosis and meiosis (p. 1); male reproductive organs (p. 4); spermatogenesis (p. 2); differentiation of the blastocyst (p. 6); from *Human Embryology* by M. J. T. Fitzgerald, Harper's Row, Hagerstown, 1978. Immunoglobulin structure (p. 45); and cellular basis of immunity (p. 43) from Holborow, J. and Lessof, M.; Immunological mechanisms in health and disease. *Medicine International* 1981; 5: 213–220. Action of hormones (p. 42 and p. 43) from *Clinical Gynecologic Endocrinology and Infertility*: second edition. Speroff, L., Glass, R. H., Kase, N. G. Williams and Williams, Baltimore, 1978.

I am deeply indebted to Professor Alec Turnbull not only in particular for his helpful comments and for contributing a Foreword, but also for being guide, mentor and friend during the time we worked together in Oxford.

* For MRCOG Part II, by G. M. Stirrat, to be published by Churchill Livingstone in 1983

I am especially grateful to Mrs Betty French for her patience and skill in typing the manuscript.

The comments and criticisms of those using this book are sought and will be welcomed.

Bristol, 1983

G.M.S.

# Contents

# Reproductive biology

## CYTOGENETICS

### Mitosis

Process by which all somatic cells divide; involves splitting of each of the 46 chromosomes to provide a full identical (diploid) complement for both daughter cells.

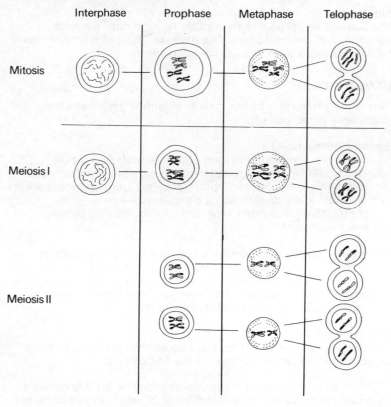

|  | Interphase | Prophase | Metaphase | Telophase |
|---|---|---|---|---|
| Mitosis |  |  |  |  |
| Meiosis I |  |  |  |  |
| Meiosis II |  |  |  |  |

1. *Interphase*: the period between successive cell division during which the cell doubles in size
2. *Prophase*: the chromatids split longitudinally into pairs of chromatids connected at the centromere
3. *Metaphase*: movement of the chromatids occurs towards the equator of the cell
4. *Telophase*: the chromatids separate and two daughter cells are formed

## Meiosis
Process by which all germ cells (gametes) divide and during which the chromosome of the daughter cells is halved (haploid).
Two sequential cell divisions are involved:
1. Interchange or crossover of chromosomal material can take place during prophase of the first division; daughter cells inherit chromatid pairs still attached at the centromere
2. Completion of separation

## Summary
The somatic cell produces by mitosis two diploid cells each containing 46 chromosomes. The germ cell by meiosis produces 4 haploid gametes each with 23 chromosomes.

## GAMETOGENESIS
This is the production of the male and female germ cells from precursors in the gonads.

### Spermatogenesis
1. Takes place in the epithelium of the seminiferous tubules
2. Germ cells (spermatogonia) begin to multiply at puberty and differentiate into primary spermatocytes; spermatogonia are diploid and divide by mitosis either into two new spermatogonia or, after repeated mitosis, into the primary spermatocytes

3. Primary spermatocytes divide into secondary spermatocytes at their first meiotic division to contain 22 + X or 22 + Y chromosomes (double-stranded except at the centromere). The second meiotic division produces spermatids with a haploid number of single-stranded chromosomes

### Spermiogenesis
The metamorphosis of spermatids into spermatozoa which takes place within the luminal border of the Sertoli cell.

　　The head of the spermatozoon, containing the DNA, is covered by a cap, the acrosome, which is the site of enzyme production to

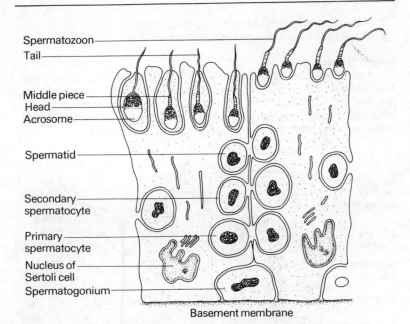

Basement membrane

allow the sperm to penetrate the ovum. The middlepiece acquires a cuff of mitochondria which provide the energy for movement. The tail consists of a central pair of fibres with an inner ring of nine fine fibres and an outer ring of nine coarse fibres.

The complete process of sperm production takes about 72 days, and each sperm is designed to carry out four tasks:

1. To 'swim' to the ovum using the energy of the mitochondria in the innerpiece
2. Orient itself to the surface of the ovum

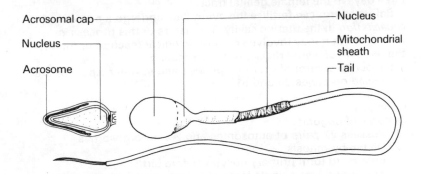

3. Activate the ovum to further development
4. Provide the paternal donation of genes

**Sperm transport**
The sperm are carried by fluid secreted by the Sertoli cells into the
rete testis and then, via the efferent ductules, to the epididymis in
the final part of which they are stored. The ability to fertilise is
obtained during passage through the epididymis but motility is not
achieved until after the sperm have left the epididymis.

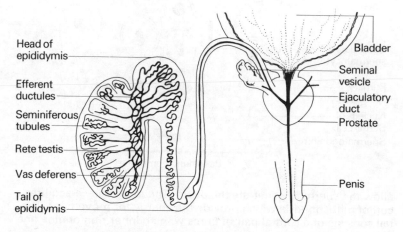

During coitus the smooth muscle of the epididymis and vas
deferens eject the sperm at ejaculation together with the seminal
plasma secreted by the seminal vesicles, prostate and
bulbourethral glands. The spermatozoa are motile within the
semen, possibly due to dilution of an epididymal inhibitory factor.
Most sperm die within 24 hours but some can survive for up to
three days in the female genital tract.

Before sperm can fertilise the ovum they undergo a process of
*capacitation* in the uterine cavity. The nature of this process is
unknown but it may involve an immunological reaction or merely
the removal of a superficial protective coating.

Endocrine control of spermatogenesis and sexual responses are
discussed on pages 36 and 51.

**Oogenesis**
Features of oogonia:
1. Possess 22 pairs of autosomes and 2 X chromosomes
2. Divide by mitosis
3. Enlarge to form primary oocytes before birth
4. Surrounded by a single layer of cells derived from the surface
   of the ovary; these are primordial follicles

Shortly before birth the primary oocytes enter the prophase of the first division of meiosis which proceeds no further until puberty. The female is born with her full stock of potential eggs but of the 200 000 or so present at birth most degenerate postnatally and only about 10 000 survive until puberty.

## Development of Graafian follicle

From the time of sexual maturity the ovary and uterus undergo monthly cyclical changes. One ovarian cycle proceeds as follows:
1. Enlargement of up to 100 follicles; the epithelial cells become columnar and the adjacent stroma form a shell or theca around them
2. The *zona pellucida* develops around the oocyte
3. One follicle ripens fully and as it grows the epithelial (granulosa) cells form the *stratum granulosum*
4. A fluid filled cavity (antrum) appears in the stratum granulosum and the whole is now called a *Graafian follicle*
5. The theca differentiates into the fibromuscular *theca externa* and the endocrine *theca interna* which produces oestrogen

## Ovulation

As the Graafian follicle matures the nucleus of the primary oocyte completes its first meiotic division and moves towards the cell surface. This division is very unequal resulting in a *secondary oocyte* and the *first polar body*. The follicle is now about 12 mm in diameter and expulsion of the secondary oocyte with its investing *corona radiata* of granulosa cells is about to occur. Shortly after ovulation the oocyte enters its second unequal meiotic division which gives rise to the ovum and the *second polar body*. This second division is not completed unless fertilisation takes place (see below). The ovum is inherently immobile and dies within 12 to 24 hours if it is not fertilised.

## Formation of the corpus luteum

1. The ruptured follicle fills with blood from torn thecal vessels
2. The remaining granulosa cells enlarge and produce *progesterone*.
3. The cells of the *theca interna* also enlarge and continue to secrete oestrogen.
4. The *granulosa lutein* cells and *theca lutein* cells are invaded by blood vessels to complete the formation of the corpus luteum by the fourth post-ovulatory day

If fertilisation does not occur the corpus luteum undergoes rapid degeneration after 10 days. Ultimately only a pale scar, the *corpus albicans* remains in the ovarian cortex.

If the ovum is fertilised and implantation occurs the corpus luteum persists and enlarges.

The hypothalamo-pituitary control of the ovarian and menstrual cycle are discussed on pages 31 and 32.

## EMBRYOLOGY

### 1. Fertilisation

(i) At ovulation the ovum is deposited near the fimbrial end of the fallopian tube

(ii) Entry into the tube occurs due to the fimbrial ciliated epithelium

(iii) Of the millions of sperm deposited in the vagina, only a few thousand enter the fallopian tubes and of these only a few hundred reach the ovum. Many of these penetrate the cells of the corona radiata due to the release of hyaluronidase from the acrosome in the head of the spermatozoon

(iv) The corona radiata cells detach from the zona pellucida and one another after fertilisation which usually takes place in the ampulla (i.e. outer third) of the tube

(v) Movement of the sperm on the zona pellucida causes the ovum to rotate and this may facilitate tubal transport

(vi) Many sperm pierce the zona pellucida to enter the *perivitelline space* but only one sperm can pierce the *vitelline membrane*

(vii) The whole spermatozoon is engulfed but the neck and tail become detached from the head and disintegrate. The head now forms the *male pronucleus*

(viii) Penetration of the vitelline membrane causes the second meiotic division of the oocyte to be completed. The second polar body is extruded into the perivitelline space (where, rarely, it may itself be fertilised). The ovum is now termed the *female pronucleus*

(ix) The male and female pronuclei fuse to form the *zygote* and restore the normal diploid number of chromosomes

### 2. Formation of the blastocyst

The zygote becomes the morula and then the blastocyst by repeated cell division or cleavage.

| Event | Time from fertilisation |
|---|---|
| First cleavage | 30 hours |
| Second cleavage | 40 hours |
| Morula formed (16 cell stage to formation of blastocyst) | 50 to 60 hours |
| Morula reaches uterus and blastocyst forms (from 50 to 60 cell stage) | 4 to 5 days |
| Implantation begins | 7 days |
| Implantation is complete | 14 days |

The morula differentiates into two cell groups:

(i) The *trophoblast* which invades the uterine wall and establishes the placenta

(ii) The *embryoblast* which produces all the tissues of the embryo from three different cellular layers — the ectoderm, the mesoderm and the endoderm (see below)

## 3. Implantation and development of the placenta
(i) The blastocyst always implants at its *embryonic pole* where embryoblast meets trophoblast
(ii) Implantation occurs on the posterior wall in about two-thirds of cases and on the anterior wall in about one third of cases

The timetable is as follows:

| Days from fertilisation | |
|---|---|
| 7 | (First day of implantation) |
| | (i) Flat-celled trophoblast gives rise to cytotrophoblast which is itself the origin of syncytiotrophoblast |
| | (ii) Maternal capillaries enlarge and multiply |
| | (iii) Endometrium undergoes decidual reaction commencing at implantation site and spreading throughout endometrium in a few days |
| 8 | Syncytiotrophoblast begins to erode maternal sinusoids |
| 12 | (i) Embryoblast and trophoblast cooperate to form the amniotic and yolk sacs which are contiguous. |
| | (ii) Extra-embryonic mesoderm has developed |
| | (iii) Nidation is almost complete |
| | (iv) Lacunae develop in which trophoblast is in direct contact with maternal blood. (A little vaginal bleeding may occur causing confusion over date of L.M.P.) |
| | (v) Cytotrophoblast forms cell columns within the invading syncytiotrophoblast to form *primary villi* |
| 14 | (i) Syncytiotrophoblast spreads radially |
| | (ii) Cytotrophoblast columns push through the syncytium and merge to form the *cytotrophoblast shell* surrounding the whole conceptus |
| | (iii) The cytotrophoblast shell is pierced by maternal sinusoids as they become lacunae which have coalesced to form the intervillous space |
| | (iv) Secondary villi develop an extra embryonic mesoderm as they enter the cytotrophoblast columns |
| 16 | (i) The cytotrophoblast shell is well developed. |
| | (ii) Blood vessels are differentiating from the chorionic mesoderm which extend into the secondary villi to form the *tertiary villi* |
| | (iii) Each villus is supplied by one fetal artery and drained by one fetal vein |
| 14—21 | (i) The conceptus begins to encroach on the uterine cavity |
| | (ii) It is completely surrounded by decidua |
| | (iii) That on the maternal side is the *decidua basalis* |
| | (iv) The *decidua capsularis* is on the side nearest the cavity |

*The timetable continued*

*Days from*
*fertilisation*

|  | | |
| --- | --- | --- |
|  | (v) | The *decidua parietalis* covers the remainder of the uterine cavity |
|  | (vi) | The decidua basalis and capsularis gradually fuse and obliterate the cavity |
| 21–28 | (i) | The fetal circulation becomes established and feto-maternal interchange begins |
|  | (ii) | Fetal and maternal blood are separated at all times by fetal capillary endothelium and by trophoblast |

## 4. Phases of development of the conceptus
  (i) The ovum — from fertilisation to implantation (two weeks)
 (ii) The embryo — organogenesis occurs as the definitive placenta develops (weeks three to eight)
(iii) The fetus — primarily a time of maturation and increasing size (weeks nine to term)

## 5. General aspects of development of embryo and membranes up to day 14 after fertilisation
  (i) The embryoblast begins to differentiate into two apposed discoid groups of cells, the *ectoderm* and *endoderm*, as implantation is progressing

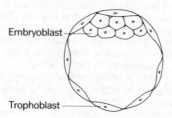

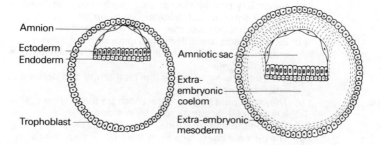

(ii) The first somite appears at the junction of the primitive brain and spinal cord on day 20. By day 30, 28 somites have appeared

(iii) The mesoderm beside the cephalic portion of the neural plate (the brain plate) does not segment and it is in this tissue that the *branchial arches* develop

(iv) The first pair to appear are the *mandibular arches*

(v) Another two pairs appear by the end of the third week which come between the mandibular arches and the developing heart. A further two pairs develop later

(vi) No segmentation occurs in the mesoderm lateral to the somites close to which is the *intermediate mesoderm*

(vii) External to this is the *lateral plate mesoderm* in which lies the embryonic coelom, and which is divided into somatic (against the amnion) and splanchnic (against the yolk sac) mesoderm

(viii) The somatic mesoderm with its related amnion is known as the *somatopleure*

(ix) The splanchnic mesoderm and related yolk sac endoderm form the *splanchnopleure*

(x) From the somites develop the trunk muscles, and the vertebral column

(xi) The intermediate mesoderm will produce the kidneys, adrenal cortex and gonads

(xii) Limb buds grow from the lateral plate mesoderm

**9. Formation of the neural tube**

(i) As the paraxial mesoderm thickens the neural plate overlying it becomes folded

(ii) Gradually the neural folds meet to form the neural tube, in which neurectoderm and skin ectoderm from one side fuse with neurectoderm and skin ectoderm from the other side

(iii) These two elements then separate so that the neural tube lies ventral to the skin ectoderm

(iv) Fusion of the folds begins at the level of the earlier somites and proceeds both cephalad and caudally

(v) The upper and lower open ends of the neural tube are the *neuropores*

(vi) As the neural folds are about to fuse, cells at the crest of the neurectoderm escape and form the *neural crest* lying dorsal and lateral to the closed neural tube

(vii) The continuing segmentation of the mesoderm into somites breaks up the neural crest into individual cell groups which will ultimately form the:
a. Dorsal root ganglia
b. Sheaths of peripheral nerves
c. Ganglia of the autonomic nervous system
d. Chromaffin tissue (including the adrenal medulla)

  e. Melanoblasts and
  f. Cartilage within the branchial arches

## 10. The effects of embryonic folding on amniotic and yolk sacs
  (i) The amniotic sac expands rapidly and the embryo becomes
       completely enclosed in and protected by amniotic fluid
  (ii) When flexion folding is complete the embryo is entirely
       covered by skin ectoderm which later becomes the epidermis
 (iii) The yolk sac is constricted by the body folds becoming
       pinched like an hour glass
 (iv) That portion of the yolk sac retained within the embryo will
       become the gut while the extra-embryonic portion regresses
       and cannot usually be identified at birth
  (v) The connection between the gut and yolk sac remnant is the
       *vitelline duct*
 (vi) The embryonic *foregut* extends from that point up to the oral
       membrane. It thus includes the future pharynx and
       oesophagus which are not considered to be 'gut' structures in
       the adult
(vii) The *midgut* is opposite the vitelline duct
(viii) The *hindgut* continues caudally to the *cloacal membrane*
 (ix) The *cloaca* is the part of the hindgut caudal to the allantois

## 11. The cardiovascular system
  (i) The embryonic blood vessels tend to form in plexuses which
       provides alternative channels and allows the most appropriate
       to develop. (This explains the variations in the vascular system
       found in the adult)
  (ii) A capillary plexus develops which communicates with the
       vitelline vessels
 (iii) The heart develops from the splanchnic mesoderm and begins
       to beat about 21 days following fertilisation
 (iv) Initially it is only a primitive heart tube from which blood
       passes to an aortic sac, through the branchial arches and into
       the dorsal aortae
  (v) Some blood goes to the brain via the internal carotid arteries
       but the majority passes through three major plexuses
       a. The vitelline vessels to the yolk sac and gut
       b. The intersegmental arteries and cardinal veins to supply the
          nervous system and body wall
       c. The umbilical vessels to the placenta
These have developed by day 24.

## 12. Blood formation
  (i) Blood islands develop on the surface of the yolk sac which
       contain the stem cells of the red and white cells of the blood

(ii) Erythropoiesis begins in the liver (and to a small extent in the spleen) during the sixth week from conception and reaches its peak at about 16 weeks. Bone marrow erythropoiesis begins at about 16 weeks

(iii) Granulocytes develop from stem cells which migrate from yolk sac to bone marrow and can be found in the circulation from the tenth week

(iv) Lymphocytes develop in the thymus from nine weeks and in the lymph nodes from 10 weeks

## 13. The kidneys and ureters

Three successive systems develop, the *pronephros, mesonephros* and the *metanephros*. The last is the definitive kidney in man.

(i) The pronephros develops in the cervical region

(ii) As it wanes the mesonephros appears in the thoraco-lumbar intermediate mesoderm

(iii) Renal tubules develop which open into the pronephric duct which now becomes the *mesonephric duct* opening into the cloaca

(iv) Near the point at which this duct enters the cloaca the *ureteric bud* develops from the dorsal aspect of the duct and it extends into the intermediate mesoderm

(v) The bud develops a lumen to form the *ureter* then the *renal pelvis*

(vi) The ureteric bud divides and branches progressively to form the calyceal system and collecting tubules

(vii) Cells from the surrounding intermediate mesoderm contribute the *metanephric cap* which differentiate into nephrons comprising Bowman's capsule, a proximal convoluted tubule, the loop of Henlé and a distal convoluted tubule (which opens into a collecting tubule)

(viii) Bowman's capsule is invaginated by a capillary tuft to complete the system

(ix) The kidneys lie in front of the sacrum at first but they have ascended to their adult position by the end of the eighth week from conception

## 14. The bladder and urethra

(i) The hindgut and allantois open into a common endodermal chamber, the cloaca

(ii) A mesodermal septum grow into it caudally to meet the cloacal membrane and splitting the cloaca into a ventral *urogenital sinus* and the dorsal *rectum*

(iii) The mesonephric ducts open into the urogenital sinus and above their point of entry the urogenital sinus expands to form the *primitive bladder*

(iv) The allantois regresses leaving the vestigial urachus linking the fundus of the bladder to the umbilicus
(v) The primitive bladder in time incorporates the lower ends of the mesonephric ducts so that the ureters open into it
(vi) The definitive *bladder* is completed by the development of a muscle coat from the surrounding mesoderm
(vii) The openings of the mesonephric ducts are carried down to form the urethra

## 15. Gonadal development — early stages
(i) The earliest stages of testicular and ovarian development are indistinguishable
(ii) Germ cells arise probably from yolk sac endoderm early in the development of the embryo
(iii) They travel from the yolk sac close to the allantois to the intermediate mesoderm
(iv) During the fifth week of development the epithelium on the coelomic surface of the intermediate mesoderm develops into the *germinal epithelium* (named when it was thought to give rise to germ cells)
(v) The *sex cords* grow from the germinal epithelium into the mesoderm and the germ cells migrate along the cords to take up position in both the cortex and the medulla of the gonad
(vi) The gonads are not recognisably male or female until the seventh week of development
(vii) The female gonad remains indifferent until the middle of pregnancy. The Y chromosome allows testicular differentiation

## 16. Testicular development
(i) The medullary sex cords develop further during the seventh and eighth week of gestation to form the primitive *seminiferous tubules*
(ii) The cortical germ cells and sex cords degenerate
(iii) The tubules contain interstitial (Leydig) cells and male germ cells. The former increase in number until about 24 weeks after conception and thereafter decrease markedly

## 17. Ovarian development
(i) In this case it is the cortical epithelium which develops while the medullary component regresses
(ii) The cortical sex cords invest the primary oocytes with their follicular epithelium
(iii) In mid-pregnancy placental gonadotrophin causes enlargement of the oogonia which is the stimulus for ovarian differentiation
(iv) Some sex cords may persist in the medulla until just before birth.

## 18. Genital tract development — early stages
(i) The *phallus* develops from the *genital tubercle* which derives from the mesoderm, ventral to the urogenital sinus
(ii) Epithelial buds from the sinus penetrate the surrounding mesoderm to form the glandular tissue of the *prostate* in the male and the *para-urethral glands* in the female. The bulk of the prostate is mesodermal in origin
(iii) The phallic urethra becomes an open trough as the urogenital membrane disintegrates in the seventh week. On each side are the *urogenital* and *labio-scrotal* folds
(iv) The further development of the genital tract and external genitalia is directed by the gonads
(v) Without any stimulus the genital tract would be female in form; oestrogens merely promote its growth
(vi) Androgens from the interstitial cells of the testis promote growth of the mesonephric ducts and the masculinisation of the external genitalia. They also suppress the paramesonephric ducts

## 19. Male genital tract
(i) Some of the tubules of the mesonephros are preserved in the male and they become the *efferent ductules* of the testis
(ii) The mesonephric duct becomes the *vas deferens*
(iii) The proximal part forms the epididymis
(iv) Distally it also forms the *seminal vesicle* and the *ejaculatory duct*
(v) Elongation of the male phallus forms the *penis* and the urogenital folds close to form the urethral canal
(vi) Closure of the labio-scrotal folds produces the *scrotum*
(vii) As growth of the trunk continues the testis is anchored by fibrous cord, the *gubernaculum*, which later becomes the inguinal canal
(viii) Alongside it grows a peritoneal diverticulum, the *processus vaginalis* to reach the scrotum (or labium majus)
(ix) During the last two months the testis descends along the inguinal canal and with it comes the vas deferens, and testicular vessels and nerves. The processus vaginalis is usually obliterated thereafter

## 20. Female genital tract
(i) The *paramesonephric* (Müllerian) ducts appear at five to six weeks after conception in the intermediate mesoderm as buds of coelomic epithelium at the cranial end of the urogenital ridge
(ii) Each duct grows down lateral to the mesonephric (Wolffian) duct until at a low level it crosses anterior to it and joins the paramesonephric duct from the opposite side

(iii) Fusion of the ducts begins at seven to eight weeks and is complete by 12 weeks

(iv) The lower end forms the *uterus*: the upper parts become the *fallopian tubes*.

 (v) Each paramesonephric duct is suspended from the mesonephros by a mesentery which forms a transverse partition, the *urogenital septum* between the urogenital sinus and rectum. (This is the precursor of the broad ligament)

(vi) The gubernaculum of the ovary becomes attached to the utero-tubal junction. The distal end persists as the *round ligament*; the proximal end is the *ovarian ligament*

(vii) The *vagina* forms from the *vaginal plate* at the junction of the caudal end of the paramesonephric duct where it abuts with the urogenital sinus. The plate lengthens and canalises from the vestibule upwards

(viii) The upper three-fifths of the vaginal epithelium derive from the paramesonephric epithelium while the lower two-fifths are from urogenital sinus epithelium

(ix) The *clitoris* develops from the genital tubercle

(x) The urogenital and labioscrotal folds become the *labia minora* and *majora* respectively

## 21. Breast development

(i) The *mammary ridge* or *milk line* extends bilaterally from the axilla to the groins from skin ectoderm in the six weeks of development

(ii) The original thickening of ectoderm remains as the nipple and downgrowths from it canalise and become the *lactiferous ducts*

(iii) Glandular acini develop from the ducts

FURTHER READING

Boyd, J. D. & Hamilton, W. J. (1970) *The Human Placenta.* Heffer: Cambridge

Fitzgerald, M. J. T. (1978) *Human Embryology*. Harper and Row: Hagerstown

Hamilton, W. J., Boyd, J. D. & Mossman, H. W. (1972) *Human Embryology.* Heffer: Cambridge

## ANATOMY

This section covers details of anatomy of relevance in obstetrics and gynaecology.

### The hypothalamus

Part of the diencephalon at the base of the brain, forming the floor of the third ventricle and part of its lateral walls.

Within it are cells which share characteristics of both neurones and endocrine gland cells secreting trophic hormones (see p. 37).

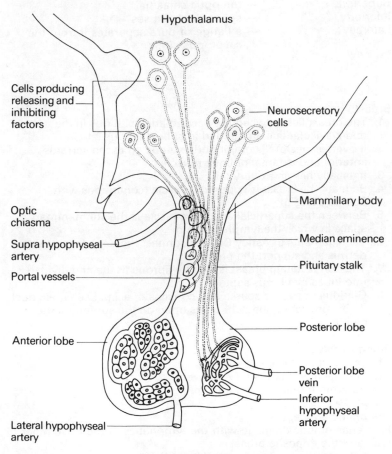

Hypothalamus

Cells producing releasing and inhibiting factors

Neurosecretory cells

Optic chiasma

Mammillary body

Supra hypophyseal artery

Median eminence

Portal vessels

Pituitary stalk

Posterior lobe

Anterior lobe

Posterior lobe vein

Inferior hypophyseal artery

Lateral hypophyseal artery

Pituitary

## Pituitary gland

Lies in the *sella turcica* in the middle cranial fossa.

*Blood supply*
1. Anterior pituitary supplied by a portal system originating in capillaries of the median eminence of the hypothalamus. The flow is from brain to pituitary. No nervous connection exists between the brain and pituitary so neuro-chemical transmitters must travel in the portal circulation.
2. Posterior pituitary supplied by the internal carotid artery

*Anatomical relations*

| | |
|---|---|
| Superiorly | — the optic chiasma |
| Inferiorly | — sphenoidal sinuses |
| Laterally | — a flange of dura separates it from the cavernous sinus. |

## Breast

1. The breast lies between the second and sixth ribs in the mid-clavicular line embedded in subcutaneous fat
2. It overlies pectoralis major and extends on to the serratus anterior and external oblique muscles
3. It usually has an axillary tail
4. Beneath the breast is superficial fascia (continuous with Scarpa's fascia)
5. Between the superficial and deep fascia is the submammary space in which the lymphatics run
6. The ligaments of Astley Cooper connect the deep fascia to the dermis and support the breast
7. The non-lactating breast is mainly fibrous tissue and divided into lobes by fibrous septa
8. Glandular tissue is sparse and consists of acini. Each main duct drains one lobe. About 15 ducts open on the summit of the nipple

*Blood supply*
1. Lateral thoracic artery and vein
2. Internal mammary artery and vein
3. Acromio-thoracic artery and vein

*Lymphatic drainage*
Free anastomotic drainage with the lymphatics of the abdominal wall and the opposite breast.
   A *subareolar plexus* drains the superficial parts of the breast.
   A *submammary* plexus drains the deep parts as shown.

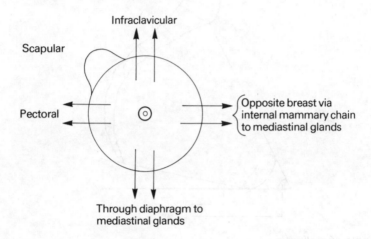

Infraclavicular

Scapular

Pectoral

Opposite breast via
internal mammary chain
to mediastinal glands

Through diaphragm to
mediastinal glands

## The bony pelvis
Divided into false and true pelvis by an oblique plane through the
sacral promontory and the arcuate line laterally and anteriorly.
   The true pelvis has an inlet and cavity and an outlet.
   The pelvic inlet has three principal diameters.
1. *Antero-posterior or true conjugate* — from the sacral
   promontory to the upper border of the symphysis pubis
   Average measurement — 11.0 cm
2. *Oblique* — from the iliopubic eminence to the opposite
   sacro-iliac joint
   Average measurement — 12.5 cm
3. *Transverse* — from the middle of the brim on one side to the
   same point on the other
   Average measurement — 13.5 cm
   The *cavity* is a short curved canal bounded
     (i) In front and below by the pubic rami and symphysis
    (ii) Above and behind by the sacrum and coccyx
   (iii) Laterally by the pelvic surfaces of the ilium and ischium
   The *outlet* is bounded behind by the tip of the coccyx and
laterally by the ischial tuberosities separated by the pubic arch
anteriorly and the bilateral sciatic notches.

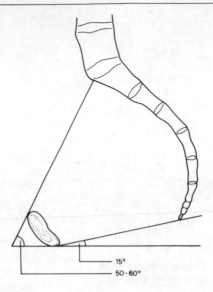

*Angle of inclination*

*Differences between male and female pelvis*
The female pelvis is a short section of a long cone. The male pelvis
is a long section of a short cone.

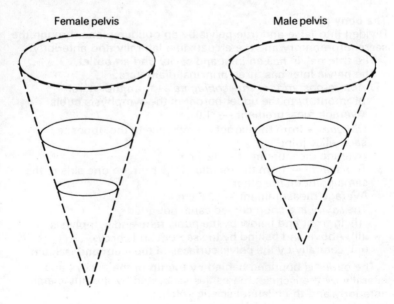

## Pelvic wall muscles

*1. Obturator internus muscle*

Origins:  obturator membrane
        bony margin of obturator foramen
        across ischium to greater sciatic notch

Inserted into medial surface of greater trochanter by passing through the lesser sciatic foramen.

Nerve supply: nerve to obturator internus (L5; S1, 2)

Points: The obturator nerve and vessels pass through the area of the obturator foramen not filled by the obturator membrane.


*2. Piriformis muscle*

Origins:   middle three pieces of sacrum
         adjoining lateral mass

Insertion: upper border of greater trochanter by passing
         through the greater sciatic notch.

Nerve supply: $S_1$ and $S_2$.

Points: The emerging sacral nerves and sacral plexus lie on its surface.


## The pelvic foor

The pelvic floor is a gutter-shaped sheet of muscle slung around the midline structures. The gutter slopes downwards and forwards.

The investing muscles are together known as the *levatores ani* and they comprise:

*1. Ischio-coccygeus*

Origin:         the tip of the ischial spine
Insertion:      lowest piece of the sacrum side of the coccyx
Nerve supply:  the perineal branch of S4

Points: Its gluteal surface is the sacro-spinous ligament. It lies edge-to-edge with piriformis.


*2. Ilio-coccygeus*

Origin:         the posterior part of the arcus tendineus (see
             below)
Insertion:      side of the coccyx
             the ano-coccygeal raphé (see below)
Nerve supply:  the perineal branch of S4

Points: The levatores ani muscles originally arose from the pelvic brim but migration has occurred down the pelvic side wall and each *arcus tendineus* (white line) was brought with the muscles.

The *ano-coccygeal raphé* is an interdigitation of fibres of right and left levatores ani running from the tip of the coccyx to the junction of the rectum and the anal canal.

### 3. Pubo-coccygeus

Origins:          anterior half of the arcus tendineus posterior
                  surface of the body of the pubis

Insertion:        tip of coccyx and ano-coccygeal raphé
                  fibres from the pubis swing round the ano-rectal
                  junction and join fibres from the opposite side
                  (with some fibres from pubo-rectalis)
                  the perineal body as a muscular sling behind the
                  vagina

Nerve supply:     inferior haemorrhoidal nerves
                  perineal nerves

## Blood supply of pelvic structures

### 1. Arterial supply

The *common iliac artery* bifurcates at the sacro-iliac joint into external and internal iliac arteries.

The *internal iliac artery* has posterior and anterior divisions.

The *posterior division* has three branches which supply parietal structures:

(i)  ilio-lumbar artery
(ii) superior gluteal artery
(iii) lateral sacral artery

The *anterior division* has three parietal and four visceral branches.

**parietal branches:**

(i)  Inferior gluteal artery
(ii) Internal pudendal artery
(iii) Obturator artery — a small branch anastomoses with the pubic branch of the inferior epigastric artery and this forms the abnormal obturator artery in 30 per cent of cases

**visceral branches:**

(i)  Superior vesical artery (the canalised proximal end of the lateral umbilical artery); supplies the bladder
(ii) Inferior vesical artery; supplies the trigone and the ureter.
(iii) Uterine artery
(iv) Vaginal artery (may branch from the uterine)

### 2. Venous return

Each pelvic viscus drains into a venous plexus around it.

(i)   Uterine and rectal plexus drain to the internal iliac veins
(ii)  Ovarian (pampiniform) plexus drains to the inferior vena cava on the right and the renal vein on the left
(iii) Veins corresponding to the parietal branches of the divisions of the internal iliac artery drain to the internal iliac veins
(iv)  The visceral plexuses of one side anastomose with those of the other and with Batson's external vertebral plexus

**Nerve supply of pelvic structures**
Obturator nerve (L2,3,4) — nerve of adductor compartment of thigh.

Sacral plexus L4 and 5 form the *lumbo-sacral trunk* which crosses over the ala of the sacrum and descends to join S1-4 to form the sacral plexus resting on piriformis and covered by pelvic fascia.

The sacral plexus has six branches:
1. The pudendal nerve (S2,3,4) which passes between piriformis and ischio-coccygeus, curls around the sacro-spinous ligament to enter the ischio-rectal fossa
2. The pelvic splanchnics (S2,3)
3. Twigs to piriformis
4. Posterior cutaneous nerve of the thigh
5. Perforating cutaneous nerve
6. Perineal branch of S4

**The ovary**
1. Lies on the peritoneal side wall of the pelvis in the angle between the internal and external vessels on the obturator nerve
2. It is attached to the posterior leaf of the broad ligament by the *mesovarium* which does not invest the ovary

The *ovarian or infundibilo pelvic ligament* is a fibro-muscular structure between the layers of the broad ligament which is a residual of part of the gubernaculum (see p. 15)

*Blood supply*: the ovarian artery is a branch of the aorta arising just below the renal artery.

A pampiniform plexus in the mesovarium and infundibilo-pelvic ligament drains to the ovarian veins which accompany the ovarian artery except that the left ovarian vein drains to the left renal vein.

Ovarian cycle — see page 33.

**The uterus**
The uterus has three anatomical sections
1. *Fundus* lying above the insertion of the tubes
2. *Body*
3. *Cervix*

*Blood supply*: the *uterine artery*, a branch of the anterior division of the internal iliac artery:
(i) Passes medially across the pelvic floor in the base of the broad ligament above the ureter
(ii) Reaches the uterus at the supravaginal part of the cervix where it gives off a branch to the cervix and vagina
(iii) Turns upwards within the leaves of the broad ligament to the

entrance of the tubes where it anastomoses end-to-end with
the tubal branch of the ovarian artery

The myometrium and endometrium are supplied as follows:

Myometrial arcuate arteries become radial arteries

Endometrial spiral and basal arteries

Venous return is through the plexus in the broad ligament which
joins with the vesical and rectal plexuses and pass to the internal
iliac vein.

*Lymphatic drainage*

Body: internal iliac glands

Cervix:  internal iliac and obturator glands

Nerve supply: The motor pathways are not known. Pain from the
cervix passes in the *nervi erigentes* (S2,3). The body nerve supply
is by the lumbar splanchnics to the lower thoracic segments.

*Uterine structure*

The myometrium consists of smooth muscle cells grouped into
bundles separated by connective tissue. The muscle bundles are in
several layers

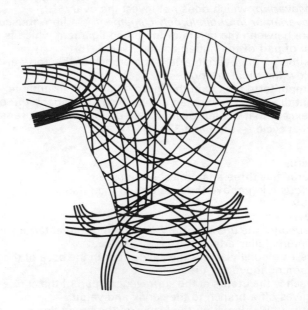

Innermost longitudinal
Vascular layer with bundles in all directions
Outermost circular and longitudinal layers
The last merge into the cervix and ligamentous supports of the uterus. There is a gradual fall in smooth muscle content from the fundus to the cervix: 80 per cent of the non-pregnant cervix is collagen and only 10 per cent is muscle.

## Bladder
The bladder has two main anatomical areas:

1. *Trigone*
    (i) A triangular area between the urethra and ureteric orifices (the ureteric bar)
    (ii) The ureters pierce it obliquely which provides a sphincteric action
    (iii) It is fixed by the lateral ligaments of the bladder, the cervix and the anterior fornix of the vagina

2. *Fundus*
    (i) Lies behind the symphysis pubis with the retropubic space or cave, of Retzius between them
    (ii) Held in position by the fixed trigone assisted by the umbilical ligaments and the pelvic peritoneum. The muscular wall is the *detrusor* muscle with fibres running in many directions
    *Blood supply*: superior and inferior vesical arteries. The venous vesical plexus communicates with the veins at the base of the broad ligament and then the internal iliac veins.
    *Nerve supply*: sympathetic supply comes from the pelvic plexuses which are inhibitory to the detrusor, and motor to the internal urethral sphincter.
    Parasympathetic supply is by the nervi erigentes.

## The ureter
1. Passes down on psoas muscle, crosses the genito-femoral nerve, and leaves psoas at the bifurcation of the common iliac artery over the sacro-iliac joint
2. For the second half of its length it lies in contact with the peritoneum of the pouch of Douglas to the level of the ischial spine
3. It then passes forward across the pelvic floor in loose areolar tissue to the bladder
4. The uterine artery is the only structure to pass between it and the pelvic peritoneum
5. It is narrowed at three points: the pelvi-ureteric junction, the pelvic brim at the sacro-iliac joint, and the bladder

6. Viewed at excretion urography the ureter can normally be seen to:
   (i) Run level with the tips of the transverse processes of the lumbar vertebrae
   (ii) Cross the sacro-iliac joint
   (iii) Run to the ischial spines and then, foreshortened, to the pubic tubercle
7. *Blood supply*:
   upper part — renal artery and vein
   middle part — ovarian artery and vein
   lower part — inferior and superior
     vesical artery and internal iliac vein.

## The urethra

The urethra, about 4 cm long in the adult, consists predominantly of two layers of muscle; an inner longitudinal layer and an outer semicircular coat, both of which are continuations of muscular layers in the detrusor.

The semicircular coat is never complete, forming loops around the urethra.

There is no anatomically distinct internal sphincter but continence is maintained throughout the urethra by the semicircular coat which is in continuity with the detrusor and shares its nervous control.

As the urethra passed through the pelvic floor it becomes surrounded at its middle third by a sleeve of voluntary muscle from the anterior fibres of pubococcygeus which provides a complementary sphincter mechanism. This is aided by pubocervical fascia and 'ligaments'. This distal sphincter, though important, is relatively weak and, once the bladder neck is open, it is usually unable to withstand the high pressures brought on by coughing or movement.

### Continence in the female

The resting tone of the muscles of the above urethral sphincters creates an intraluminal pressure which occludes the urethra.

The difference between the intravesical pressure and the urethral pressure is termed 'the urethral closure pressure.'

If the closure pressure is positive (i.e. urethral > intravesical pressure) leakage of urine is virtually impossible.

The figure opposite shows that the urethra is an intra-abdominal structure until it passes through the pelvic floor muscles.

Sudden increases in intra-abdominal pressure (arrowed on the figure) such as coughing or lifting are therefore transmitted equally to bladder and upper urethra. Intravesical and urethral pressures increase to the same extent, therefore urethral closure pressure is unchanged and continence is maintained.

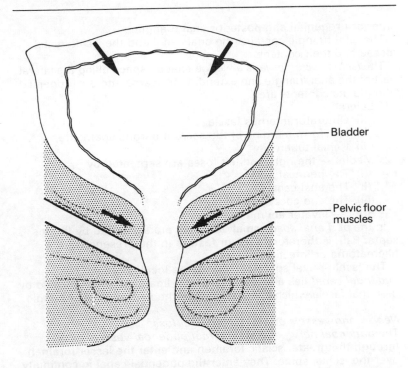

*Micturition in the female*
1. Micturition depends on the integrated function of the bladder and urethral sphincter mechanisms
2. Total bladder capacity is between 500 and 600 ml
3. First sensation is experienced at between 150 and 200 ml
4. The rise in intravesical pressure on filling, standing or coughing is < 10 cm of water
5. The bladder neck is competent in the face of sudden increases in intra-abdominal pressure despite slight loss of the posterior urethro-vesical angle and descent of the bladder base on some occasions
6. Just before or concurrent with contraction of the destrusor the urethral closure pressure falls allowing micturition to take place with minimal detrusor action
7. Voiding takes place at a maximum pressure of up to 70 cm of water with a peak flow rate of greater than 20 ml per second
8. The bladder empties entirely

**The perineum**
The perineum is that part of the pelvic outlet caudal to the pelvic diaphragm. A line joining the ischial tuberosities divides it into an

anterior urogenital and posterior anal triangle.

The anal triangle contains the anal canal and the ischio-rectal fossae and their contents.

The *ischio-rectal fossa* is a wedge-shaped space filling the lateral part of the anal triangle and extending forwards into the urogenital triangle. Its contents are:

1. Lateral
   (i) Obturator internus fascia
   (ii) Falciform margins of the sacro-tuberous ligament
   (iii) Ischial tuberosity
2. Medial — the right and left fossa are separated by
   (i) The perineal body
   (ii) The anal canal
   (iii) The ano-coccygeal body
3. Roof — levator ani muscle

In the *peri-anal space* small fat loculi are separated by fibrous septa. Pain is therefore a major feature in the presence of a haematoma or infection.

The ischio-rectal space contains large locules of fat. The *pudendal canal* lies above the falciform ligament and is formed by peri-anal fascia which splits to contain the neuro-vascular bundle.

*Nerves and vessels of the ischio-rectal fossa*

The *pudendal nerve* and the *internal pudendal vessels* pass through the greater sciatic foramen and enter the lesser foramen over the ischial spine. They enter the pudendal canal in continuity with the lesser foramen and run forwards in it to-supply the perineum.

Bartholin's glands lie beneath the fascia deep in the perineum. Their orifices lie at the middle of the lateral margins of the vaginal orifice.

FURTHER READING

Last, R. J. (1977), *Anatomy, Regional and Applied*, 6th edn. Edinburgh: Churchill Livingstone.

## HISTOLOGY

### The vagina

The vagina has three layers:

1. Outer fibrous
2. Middle muscular — outer longitudinal, inner circular
3. Stratified squamous epithelium

Epithelial papillae push deeply into the tunica propria. The vaginal skin is responsive to hormonal stimuli. Oestrogen causes the epithelial cells to be large and cornified. Without stimulation the cells are small and parabasal. In prepubertal children and postmenopausal women the epithelium is thin because of a relative lack of stimulation by oestrogen.

## The cervix
The cervix too has three distinct histological features:
1. (i) Ectocervix is stratified squamous
     a. Non-cornified
     b. Papillae less well marked than vagina
   (ii) Endocervix changes abruptly to tall and cylindrical picket cells
2. Racemose glands (i.e. like a bunch of grapes) which produce cervical mucus
3. Stroma — dense connective tissue with spindle cells. Basement membrane marks the junction between the epithelium and stroma. Muscle cells appear towards the internal os

## The endometrium
A specialised form of connective tissue characterised by its remarkable lability, regenerative capacity and sensitivity to ovarian hormones.
The endometrium is divided into:
1. A *superficial layer* with an upper spongy zone and a compact area. These are the only zones responsive to the biphasic hormonal stimulus
2. A *basal layer* of undifferentiated cells which show only oestrogenic effects even premenstrually. Histology at different phases of menstrual cycle
1. *Postmenstrual* (about one week after the end of menstrual flow).
    (i) The endometrium is thin
    (ii) The surface epithelium is low cuboidal
    (iii) The glands are straight
    (iv) The stroma is dense, compact (with little cytoplasm and large, dark, round nuclei) and non-vascular
2. *Interval phase* (one week after menses to two weeks before next)
    (i) In the early interval (pre-ovulatory) phase the epithelium proliferates and then secretory changes supervene
    (ii) The stroma becomes more abundant and hyperaemic
   *Note*: It is not possible to date an endometrium with absolute accuracy merely by histology because there is considerable variation among women.
3. *Premenstrual phase*
    (i) The endometrium is up to 8 mm thick
    (ii) The surface epithelium is tall, non-secretory;
    (iii) The glands are very tortuous

(iv) The glandular epithelium shows different features at each level
   a. Superficial compact layer — abundant stroma between glands
   b. Middle spongy layer — glands most tortuous; the epithelium is low, pale and the nuclei are at the basement membrane
   c. Basal layer — no secretory response at all
(v) Basal and spiral arterioles are prominent
(vi) Shortly before menstruation polymorph and round cell infiltration begins

*Note*: It is impossible to distinguish advanced progestational endometrium from that in early pregnancy unless chorionic villi can be seen.

4. *Bleeding phase*
   (i) Vasoconstriction of the spiral vessels causing ischaemia
   (ii) Subsequent vasodilatation brings about haemorrhage into and desquamation of the tissues
   (iii) The compact and spongy layers are lost completely by the third day

The epithelium regenerates from the stumps of glands in the basal layer. It begins even as the desquamation is occurring and the surface is re-epithelialised very quickly.

5. *The endometrium in pregnancy* (*decidua*).
   (i) The epithelium is low, pale and secretory
   (ii) The glands show saw-tooth convolutions and scalloping
   (iii) Later the glands tortuosity lessens but the epithelium becomes even flatter
   (iv) The stromal cells are larger, polygonal and arranged in a mosaic

In the spongy layer the glandular hypertrophy and convolutions are most marked. The basal layer stands out in very sharp contrast.

## Fallopian tubes

The fallopian tube is in four portions
1. Interstitial — traversing the muscle of the cornu
2. Isthmic — adjacent to the uterus
3. Ampulla — widened middle third
4. Infundibulum — the remainder including the fimbriae

It has three layers
1. Outer serous peritoneum
2. Muscular
   (i) Inner circular
   (ii) Outer longitudinal
   (iii) Incomplete longitudinal layer at the uterine end
3. Mucous membrane — the endosalpinx lies in longitudinal folds or rugae; there are only three to four at the proximal end but they have branched and divided repeatedly by the fimbrial end

There are three cells types in the mucous membrane.
1. Ciliated cells
   (i) Develop most rapidly in the interval phase
   (ii) The cilia are long, attached to a layer of basal granules
   (iii) They propel the ova and keep the tubal lumen clean
2. Non-ciliated cells have a secretory function
   (i) Their cytoplasm is extruded into the lumen
   (ii) Despite this and the need for regeneration no mitoses are seen in tubular epithelium
3. Peg cells like long, dark rods squeezed between adjoining cells. They represent a phase in the life-cycle of secretory cells

FURTHER READING

Macdonald, R. R. (ed.) (1978) *Scientific Basis of Obstetrics and Gynaecology*, 2nd edn. Edinburgh: Churchill Livingstone
Sherman, R. P. (ed.) (1979) *Human Reproductive Physiology*, 2nd edn. Oxford: Blackwells
Speroff, L., Glass, H. & Kase, N. G. (1978) *Clinical Gynecologic Endocrinology and Infertility.* Baltimore: Williams and Wilkins
Tyson, E. H. (ed.) (1978) Neuroendocrinology of reproduction. *Clinics in Obstetrics and Gynaecology*, Vol. 5, No. 2. London: W. B. Saunders.

## FERTILITY IN THE FEMALE

### The hypothalamus
Controls anterior pituitary function by substances secreted by cells within it and transported to the pituitary *via* the portal circulation (see p. 17).
1. A single decapeptide neurotransmitter controls FSH and LH-gonadotrophin releasing hormone (GnRH). Its half-life is only a few minutes and a continuous but variable release occurs. Release is controlled by
   (i) A long feedback loop due to circulating target gland hormones
   (ii) A short feedback loop due to the effect of gonadotrophins on the hypothalamus
   (iii) An ultrashort feedback by which it inhibits its own synthesis
   (iv) A series of neurotransmitters such as serotonin, melatonin, noradrenaline and dopamine (see below)
   The hypothalamus exerts a negative control on prolactin through *prolactin inhibitory factor* which is thought to be dopamine synthesised by nerve terminals from tyrosine via dihydrophenylalanine (DOPA).

*The pituitary gland* — it is influenced by the hypothalamus via the following pathways:
1. *Tonic and cyclic centres for the secretion of* GnRh
   (i) The tonic centre is responsible for basal levels of gonadotrophin. Oestradiol has a negative feedback effect on it and it is also dopamine-dependent. It is situated in the medial basal hypothalamus
   (ii) The cyclic centre is responsive to positive feedback by oestradiol and produces the mid-cycle surge of gonadotrophins. It lies in the pre-optic area in the anterior part of the hypothalamus
2. *Tancytes* — specialised ciliated ependymal cells which line the third ventricle and terminate on the portal vessels. They can therefore transport substances from, for example, the pineal gland, via the ventricular CSF to the portal circulation. They alter in response to steroids and during the ovarian cycle
3. *The posterior pituitary pathway*
   (i) Cells in the supraoptic and paraventricular nuclei secrete vasopressin, oxytocin and neurophysin
   (ii) They are transported along the pituitary stalk to the posterior pituitary where they are stored in axonal terminals
   (iii) They also pass into the CSF and then to the portal system of the anterior pituitary
   (iv) Vasopressin may assist in ACTH and growth hormone secretion
   (v) Oxytocin may be involved in gonadotrophin secretion
   (vi) Two neurophysins have been identified; one (nicotine neurophysin) is involved with vasopressin; the other (oestrogen neurophysin) accompanies oxytocin

**Gonadotrophin release**
There are two pools, one released immediately it is synthesised and the other held in reserve.
   (i) The rate of storage exceeds release which makes the mid-cycle surge possible. (This is also the time when sensitivity to GnRh is greatest)
   (ii) Oestradiol inhibits immediate release and increases storage
   (iii) This effect is overcome by the positive feedback action of oestradiol on the cyclic centre
   (iv) Low levels of progesterone increase release and storage after oestrogen priming

**Regulation of the menstrual cycle**
*Initial follicular growth (days 2–6)*
   1. Initiation of follicular growth is independent of gonadotrophin stimulation

2. Follicles grow during infancy, ovulation, periods of anovulation, pregnancy and the menopause until the numbers are exhausted
3. For the vast majority of follicles growth is limited and atresia inevitable
4. As FSH levels increase a group of follicles begins to grow further but the mechanism by which these follicles is chosen is unknown
5. The period of initial growth ends as oestrogen levels rise seven to eight days before the pre-ovulatory LH surge

*Mid-follicular phase (days 7–10)*
1. FSH stimulates follicular growth but also facilitates steroidogenesis by increasing the activity or number of LH receptors (Note: LH induces steroidogenesis)
2. Changes in hormonal levels are regulated by feedback mechanisms
   (i) Oestradiol inhibits FSH (negative feedback)
   (ii) Low levels of oestradiol inhibit LH
   (iii) High levels of oestradiol (>200 pg/ml sustained for about 50 hours) stimulate LH (positive feedback)

*Pre-ovulatory phase (days 10–14)*
1. Oestrogens rise slowly then rapidly to peak just before ovulation
2. FSH falls due to negative feedback
3. LH increases steadily to its mid-cycle surge
4. The follicle destined to ovulate protects itself by its own hormone production
5. Ovarian stromal cell production of androgens (androstenedione and testosterone) increases which enhances the atresia of non-ovulatory follicles and stimulates libido

*Ovulation*
1. The rapid rise in oestrogen triggers an LH surge
2. A modest rise in FSH may induce LH receptors and facilitate ovulation and luteinisation
3. The LH surge triggers resumption of meiosis by the oocyte
4. The pituitary is maximally sensitive to GnRh due to oestradiol
5. Ovulation occurs within the 24 hours of the LH surge
6. During this LH surge the secretion of GnRh and gonadotrophins is episodic
7. The end of the LH surge is partly due to
   (i) A sharp drop in plasma oestrogen levels
   (ii) The increase in progesterone
8. Degeneration of the collagen in the follicular wall allows it to rupture

9. Expulsion of the oocyte is brought about by prostaglandins induced by LH

*Luteal phase*
1. Days 1–3 post-ovulation: Granulosa cells
   (i) Increase in size
   (ii) Accumulate lutein (a yellow pigment)
   (iii) Secrete progesterone
2. Days 8–9 post-ovulation
   (i) The corpus luteum (CL) has become vascularised by a capillary network
   (ii) Peak levels of progesterone and oestradiol are reached
(A plasma level of progesterone over 15 nmol/l(5 ng/ml) is good presumptive evidence of ovulation)

3. Days 9–11 post-ovulation
   (i) The corpus luteum begins to decline unless pregnancy supervenes
   (ii) Regression may be due to a local luteolytic effect or to oestradiol production by the CL
   (iii) The normal CL requires the continuous presence of small amounts of LH
   (iv) In pregnancy it is maintained by hCG until nine to ten weeks gestation

4. In the absence of pregnancy the time from the LH surge to the menstrual flow is usually 14 days

**Puberty**
Puberty usually commences at a variable time between the ages of eight and fourteen years and takes two to four years. The typical sequence of events is:
1. Growth initiation
2. Breast development
3. Pubic hair growth
4. Onset of menses (menarche)
   The tendency towards the lowering of the age of menarche and onset of the growth spurt over recent generations due to improved nutrition and health seems to have halted. There is no particular age or size at which an individual girl can expect the menarche to occur. It is correlated with but not determined by weight. The hormonal events are as follows:
1. Before puberty the hypothalamus is very sensitive to steroids and therefore markedly suppressed due to negative feedback
2. Dehydroepiandrosterone (DHA) begins to rise between six and eight years of age; androstenedione at eight to ten years of age. However, the precise signal for pubertal changes to begin

is unknown. Oestrogen levels do not rise until ten to twelve years of age

3. Gonadotrophin secretion begins to increase due to decreasing hypothalamic sensitivity to negative feed-back signals. One of the first changes of puberty is the development of episodic LH secretions during sleep.
FSH levels plateau by mid-puberty; LH and oestradiol levels continue to rise until late puberty

4. As the sensitivity of the hypothalamus decreases sex steroids begin to induce the development of the secondary sexual characteristics

5. The positive feed-back effect of oestrogen usually develops after the menarche and may lead to anovulation in the first few cycles.

**The climacteric**

The period of time over which oestrogen levels gradually fall.

1. It starts with less frequent ovulation about the age of 40 years

2. Reaches a point at which inadequate follicular maturation and low oestrogen production causes amenorrhoea (the menopause — median age 51.4 years)

3. Ends in atrophy of secondary sex characteristics

4. Some follicles remain even after the menopause but they produce little oestrogen and are resistant to gonadotrophins

5. Elevated levels of FSH and LH indicate ovarian failure. Maximum levels of FSH (increased ten to twenty-fold) and LH (increased three-fold) are reached within one to three years of the menopause

6. Postmenopausal oestradiol levels are usually between 10 and 20 pg/ml most of which comes from peripheral conversion of testosterone and oestrone. Oestrone levels are about 30 pg/ml which is mostly derived from adrenal androstenedione

7. Ovarian production of testosterone is increased after the menopause due to gonadotrophin stimulation of ovarian stromal cells

8. The low levels of oestrogen continue to have a trophic effect on the breast, vagina and urethra

9. Ultimately the adrenal contribution becomes inadequate and ovarian secretion is negligible. Atrophy of the secondary sex characteristics follows

**FERTILITY IN THE MALE**

The testes has two functions:

1. *Steroidogenesis* by the interstitial cells of Leydig between the seminiferous tubules

2. *Spermatogenesis* which begins in the germinal epithelium of
   the tubules (see p. 2)
   The seminiferous tubules and interstitial cells are controlled by
three mechanisms:

*1. GnRH and gonadotrophins*
   (i) FSH binds to receptors in the Sertoli cells of the
       seminiferous tubules to activate adenylcyclase
  (ii) The resultant cyclic AMP activates DNA-dependent RNA
       synthesis (see p. 42)
 (iii) Androgen binding protein (ABP), androgen receptors and
       inhibin (see below) are formed within the Sertoli cells
  (iv) LH binds to specific receptors in the interstitial cells which
       triggers production of androgen and oestrogens

*2. Intratesticular modulation*
   (i) ABP transports testosterone into the seminiferous tubules
       where it is partly reduced to the much more active
       dihydrotestosterone and oestrogen. The binding protein
       allows a reservoir of androgens to develop which can be
       drawn on to stimulate spermatogenesis
  (ii) When the ABP-androgen complex reaches the epididymis
       along with the sperm the ABP is digested enzymatically
       producing a high concentration of free androgen

*3. Positive and negative feedback signals*
   (i) Testicular steroids (particularly oestrogen) inhibit GnRH
  (ii) Androgens diminish the LH releasing effect of GnRH
       without affecting FSH
 (iii) Oestrogen potentiates FSH and LH secretion by GnRH
  (iv) Seminiferous tubules secrete *inhibin*, a non-steroid
       substance, which specifically inhibits FSH release

*Effects of androgens*
The effects of androgens are:
   (i) Spermatogenesis
  (ii) Development of accessory glands
 (iii) Development of secondary sex characteristics
  (iv) Metabolic and psychic effects determining 'maleness'
   (v) Increasing sexual appetite
  (vi) Feedback on the hypothalamus and pituitary (see above)

*Erection*
Erection is due to tumescence of the penile cavernous bodies. It is
mediated through the parasympathetic nerve erigentes (S2-4)

*Ejaculation*
Ejaculation is a reflex action involving a complex coordinated

autonomic stimulation of the genital tract. It has two stages:
1. (i) Contractions of the epididymis, vas deferens and seminal vescle pump sperm from the epididymis and seminal fluid from the prostate and seminal vesicles into the posterior urethra
   (ii) As the seminal fluid arrives in the prostatic urethra contraction of the internal urethral sphincter closes the bladder neck (this prevents retrograde ejaculation)
   (iii) The second stage is triggered
2. The semen is expelled due to:
   (i) Relaxation of the external sphincter
   (ii) Rhythmic contractions of ischiocavernous, bulbo-cavernous and perineal muscles

*Testicular function and age*
Gonadal function in men is preserved well into old age and any decline is gradual.

Although FSH and LH levels remain normal, testosterone levels tend to fall suggesting decreased sensitivity to gonadotrophin.

The so-called 'male climacteric' is more likely to be related to psychological, cardiovascular and neurological effect of ageing rather than diminished production of androgens.

FURTHER READING

Lunenfeld, B. & Insler, V. (1978) *Infertility*. Berlin: Grosse Verlag.

## ENDOCRINOLOGY

A *hormone* is a substance produced by a specialised tissue which is released into the circulation, and travels to its responsive target cells upon which it exerts a characteristic effect.

**Trophic hormones**
FSH, LH, thyroid stimulating hormone (TSH) and hCG are glycoproteins comprised of two non-identical subunits bound non-covalently and designated $\alpha$ and $\beta$.

The $\beta$ subunits of all glycoprotein hormones are similar in chemical structures and interchangeable with one another. The $\beta$ subunits are characteristic for each hormone.

**Sex steroid hormones**
The basic structure of all steroid hormones is the perhydrocyclopenthane phenanthrene ring.

Relatively minor substitutions and deletions cause marked differences in biological activity.

The sex steroids are divided into three main groups according to the number of carbon atoms they contain (see figures below).

Cholesterol
(27 carbon atoms)

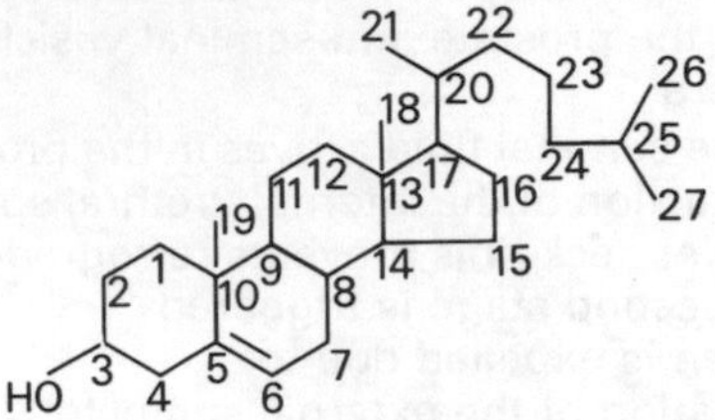

Pregnane derivatives
(21 carbon atoms) ⟶ Progestogens
                    Corticosteroids

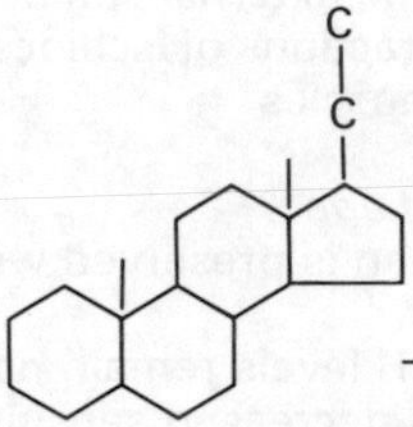

Androstane
derivatives
(19 carbon atoms) ⟶ Androgens

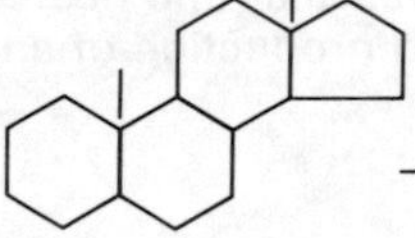

Oestrane
derivatives
(18 carbon atoms) ⟶ Oestrogens

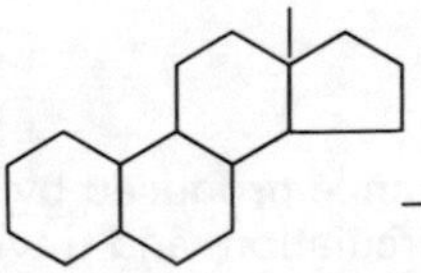

## Naming steroids

For example, testosterone is 4-Androstene-17$\beta$-ol-3-one and the structure is

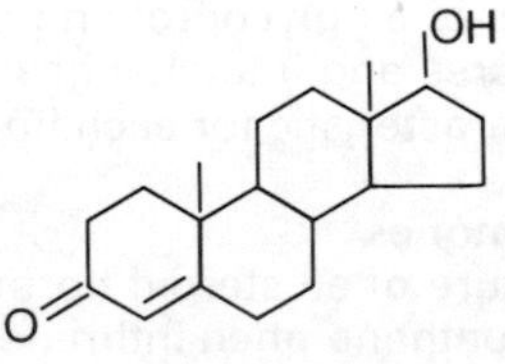

4-Androstene −17ß −ol −3 −one
(1)  (2)    (3)   (4)(8) (5) (6)   (7)

The convention for naming is:
1. The first number(s) indicates the position of any double bonds
2. The basic name follows which depends on the number of carbon atoms e.g. pregnane -21; androstane -19; oestrane -18
3. The suffix to the basic name (-ene, -drene or -triene) indicates the number (one, two or three) of double bonds
4. The next number indicates the number of the C atom(s) to which hydroxyl groups are attached
5. The following -ol, -diol, or -triol show the number (one, two, or three) of hydroxyl groups
6. The last number is the number of the C atom(s) to which ketone groups are attached
7. -one, -dione, -trione, denotes the number (one, two or three) of ketone groups
8. Almost all natural and active steroids are flat. 'Alpha' means that the substituent is below and 'beta' that it is above the plan of the ring

Among other special designations are:

Dehydro — elimination of two hydrogen atoms

Deoxy — elimination of an oxygen atom

Nor — elimination of a carbon atom

The use of delta to show the location of a double bond is outmoded.

**Steroid synthesis**
The raw material is cholesterol. The placenta is the only steroid-producing organ which cannot synthesise cholesterol from acetate. The sequence is as follows:

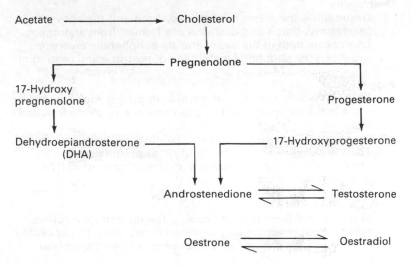

1. The selection of pathways is governed by the cell type involved.
2. During synthesis the number of carbon atoms can only be reduced, never increased
3. Conversion of cholesterol to pregnenolone takes place in mitochondria. It is a rate limiting step in the pathway and is one of the principal effects of LH
4. The ovary produces all three classes of sex steroids.
   (i) granulosa cells produce progesterone
   (ii) thecal cells produce oestrogen
   (iii) the theca with the surrounding stroma produces androstenedione, DHA and testosterone
5. The ovary lacks the 21 hydroxylase and 11 $\beta$-hydroxylase enzymes necessary to produce e.g. gluco- and mineralo-corticoids
6. The biological effects of hormones are determined by the amount of free hormone present
   (i) Most (80 per cent) of the circulating oestradiol and testosterone is bound to sex hormone binding globulin (SHBG) which is a beta globulin
   (ii) Most of the remainder is loosely bound to albumin
   (iii) Only about one per cent is free
   (iv) Progesterone, cortisol and other corticosteroids bind to a glycoprotein, corticosterone binding globulin (CBG or transcortin). About 75 per cent of cortisol is bound to CBG, 15 per cent loosely to albumin leaving 10 per cent unbound

**Oestrogens**
1. Oestradiol is the major ovarian oestrogen and the above flow chart shows that it and oestrone are formed from androgens. This occurs both in the ovary and by peripheral conversion
2. Oestriol is the peripheral metabolite of oestrone and oestradiol

**Progesterone**
1. No peripheral conversion of steroids to progesterone takes place in the non-pregnant female. There is a small contribution from the adrenal glands
2. Its metabolism is more complex than that of oestrogen. Only 10 to 20 per cent is excreted in urine as pregnanediol. Pregnanediol is the chief urinary excretion product of 17 $\alpha$ hydroxyprogesterone

**Androgen**
1. In the normal female 50 per cent of the testosterone comes from androstenedione by peripheral conversion; 25 per cent is secreted by the ovary; and 25 per cent is from the adrenal

2. Dihydrotestosterone (DHT) is the most active androgen. It is formed within the target tissues from testosterone
3. During embryonic masculine differentiation testosterone dictates the development of the mesonephric duct structures (epididymis, vas deferens and seminal vesicle). DHT is the stimulus for the urogenital sinus and tubercle to develop into the urethra, prostate and external genitalia

All steroids are excreted in urine and bile as glucuronides or sulphated conjugates.

## Mechanisms of cellular action of hormones

*Trophic hormones (e.g. GnRH, FSH, LH)*

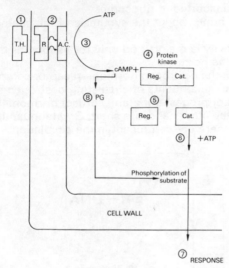

1. The trophic hormone (TH) united with a receptor (R) on the cell surface
2. Adenylate cyclase (AC) is activated
3. ATP is converted to cyclic AMP (cAMP) in the cytoplasm
4. The cAMP is bound to a cytoplasmic receptor protein which activates a protein kinase composed of regulatory (Reg.) and catalytic (Cat.) subunits
5. cAMP combines with the regulatory subunit and frees the catalytic subunit
6. Phosphorylation takes place in which phosphate is transferred from ATP to a variety of substrate proteins
7. This releases energy which triggers the appropriate physiological response

8. cAMP also stimulates prostaglandin (PG) synthesis which facilitates the response
9. In addition there may be an intracellular negative feedback mechanism involving PGs and cyclic guanosine monophosphate (cGMP)

*Sex steroids*
The most clearly defined mechanism is that for oestrogen as illustrated.
1. The hormone (E) diffuses readily across the cell membrane
2. It binds to a cytoplasmic receptor protein
3. The hormone-receptor complex crosses into the nucleus
4. It is bound to DNA
5. Messenger RNA (mRNA) is formed by gene transcription
6. mRNA is transported to ribosomes
7. Translation brings about the synthesis of the characteristic protein

Biological activity is maintained only for as long as the receptor is occupied by the hormone.

The half-life of the oestrogen hormone-receptor complex is long, therefore only small amounts of circulating oestrogen are needed.

The half-lives of progesterone and cortisol hormone-receptor complexes, on the other hand, are short. Greater quantities of each hormone must therefore be present in the circulation.

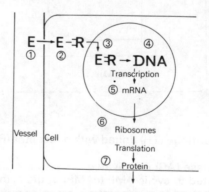

The mechanism for androgen is more complex than for oestrogens. Testosterone may be active itself or it may require intracellular conversion to dihydrotestosterone (DHT).

FURTHER READING

Speroff, L., Glass, R. H. & Kase, N. G. (1978) *Clinical Gynecologic Endocrinology and Infertility*, 2nd edn. Baltimore: The Williams and Wilkins Company.

## THE IMMUNE SYSTEM

### General considerations

The body possesses a complex system primarily based on
lymphoid cells which allows it to render harmless foreign soluble,
particulate or cellular antigens.

This immune system is equipped with many checks and balances
and none of these is more important than that which prevents
reactions against self-antigens. Auto-immune diseases arise from a
breakdown in this protective mechanism.

Once the immune system is activated it can respond by:
 (i) Producing antibody (humoral immunity)
 (ii) Developing lymphocytes which have the ability to kill foreign
      cells (cell-mediated immunity)
(iii) Recruiting other cells types
(iv) Stimulating the body's non-specific defence mechanisms (e.g.
      the inflammatory response)

After any antigen has been eliminated the system retains a
memory for it, and subsequent contact with the same antigen
results in an accelerated response.

The cellular basis and other mechanisms of the immune system
are as follows:-

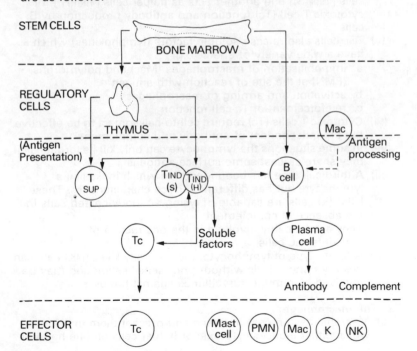

Tsup — T suppressor cell
TIND(S) — T cell which induces the production of Tsup
TIND(H) — T cells which helps B cells to produce antibody and T cells
    to become cytotoxic
Tc — cytotoxic T cell
PMN — Polymorphonuclear leucocyte
Mac — Macrophage
K — Killer cell
NK — Natural killer cell
See text for further description.

**1. The lymphocyte**
  (i) Lymphocytes arise from stem cells in the bone marrow
  (ii) There are two major types
      a. B cells, precursors of plasma cells which secrete specific
         antibody
      b. T cells which mature within the thymus and are involved in
         cell-mediated immunity
  (iii) Cellular and humoral response are regulated by inducer (TIND)
       and suppressor (Tsup) T cells
  (iv) One subpopulation of T inducer cells activates suppressor
       cells [Tsup(S)] and another acts as helper cells [TIND(H)] for
       cytotoxic T cell (Tc) function and antibody production by B
       cells
  (v) TIND cells also release soluble factors (lymphokines) which
      have a wide variety of effects e.g.
      a. immobilisation of macrophages (Mac) and polymorphs
         (PMN) at the site of reaction with antigen
      b. activation and arming of macrophages
      c. reinforcement of Tc cell function
  (vi) Cytotoxic T cells (Tc) require cell-to-cell contact to be effective
       but are independent of antibody and complement
  (vii) In some situations the lymphocyte can only kill its target cell if
        they share at least some surface antigens
  (viii) A third cell type has been identified which looks like a
         lymphocyte but has different surface characteristics. These
         killer (K) cells are capable of lysing antibody-coated cells in
         the absence of complement
         They are probably involved in the destruction of
         virus-infected cells
  (ix) A fourth type of lymphocyte, the naturally killer (NK) cell, can
       destroy tumour cells without prior sensitisation and may be
       involved in immune surveillance against tumours

**2. The macrophage**
  (i) Macrophages process antigens and present them in a form
      which either induces cytotoxic or helper cells on one hand or

suppressor cells on the other
For example, if IgG antibodies to an antigen attach themselves
to the macrophage surface that antigen is presented to the T
cell as an immune complex. This favours the production of T
suppressor cells
(ii) At a later stage in the immune reaction macrophages
phagocytose particulate antigens and antigen-antibody
complexes
(iii) They also secrete mediators of the inflammatory reaction such
as prostaglandins, complement components and hydrolytic
enzymes

## 3. Antibodies
(i) All antibodies are immunoglobulins with the following basic
structure

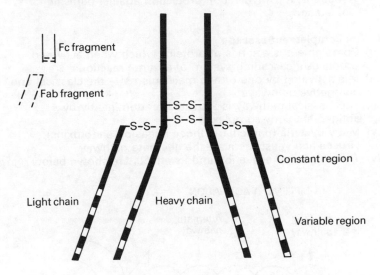

(ii) The Fc fragment has sites for e.g. complement fixation and
interaction with macrophages
(iii) The four main classes of immunoglobulin are IgA, IgG, IgM
and IgE
(iv) IgA provides surface protection at the level of the mucous
membrane. It is secreted by the mucosa-associated lymphoid
tissue (MALT) found for example in Peyer's patches, bronchial
mucosa, the breasts and genito-urinary system
(v) As paired IgA molecules pass through the mucous
membranes they acquire a glycoprotein 'secretory piece' to
become s-IgA which protects against enzymatic digestion

(vi) Colostrum is particularly rich in IgA providing passive immunity to the suckling infant

(vii) IgG is the main immunoglobulin in the plasma and has four main subclasses $IgG_1 - IgG_4$

(viii) The relatively small molecular weight of IgG (160 000) means that it can diffuse from the blood vessels into the tissues. It also crosses the placenta

(ix) $IgG_1$ and $IgG_3$ activate the complement cascade (see below)

(x) IgM is produced early in the immune response. It is a large molecule (900 000 m.w.) and tends to remain in the circulation. It does not cross the placenta

(xi) IgM circulates as a group of five immunoglobulin molecules. It is therefore a very powerful complement activator

(xii) IgE is the reaginic antibody which will bind to mast cells and basophils producing immediate allergic anaphylactic reactions. It is involved in protection against parasitic infestation

## 4. The complement cascade

(i) Complement is a series of proteins which when activated produces a cascading system of enzyme reactions

(ii) It is activated by one of two mechanisms — the classical and alternative pathways

(iii) The classical pathway is activated predominantly by antigen-antibody complexes

(iv) Many bacteria (particularly those releasing endotoxins), viruses and yeasts activate the alternate pathway

(v) The process of activation and its effects are shown below

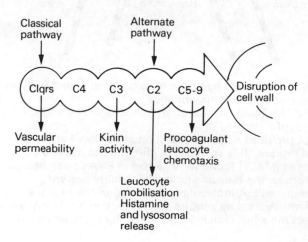

COMPLEMENT ACTIVATION

## The major histocompatibility complex (MHC)

The MHC is a system of linked genes on chromosome 6 in man which code for a series of glycoprotein surface antigens.

(i) Tissue typing has identified several of these antigens which are associated with leucocytes. They are therefore designated human leucocyte antigens (HLA)

(ii) They are, however, to be found to a varying extent on all human cells so far studied, except for villous trophoblast

(iii) Four main loci have been identified — HLA-A, -B, -C and -D. (A locus is a site on a chromosome where alternative forms of a gene (alleles) are found. Each individual can only possess a maximum of two genes at each locus i.e. one on each chromosome)

(iv) The main biological function of the major histocompatibility antigens is to regulate T-lymphocyte function. HLA-A, -B and -C participate in interactions between Tc lymphocytes and target cells. HLA-D associated antigens are found on B cells and monocytes and control the balance between helper and suppressor T cells

(v) The MHC also contain genes linked to HLA which determine susceptibility to many diseases

FURTHER READING

Roitt, I. (1980) *Essential Immunology*, 4th edn. Oxford: Blackwells.

## PROSTAGLANDINS

Prostaglandins are unsaturated fatty acids produced by all mammalian cells (with possible exception of red blood cells).

The name is derived from their discovery in human seminal fluid. Their basic structure and the numbering of their carbon atoms starting from the carboxyl group is as shown:

There are two main naturally occurring families. Each has the pentane (five membered) ring and two side chains as shown.

1. The 1 series (i.e. with *one* double bond on a side chain is derived from dihomogammalinoleic acid (DGLA)
2. The 2 series i.e. with *two* double bonds on a side chain is derived from arachidonic acid (AA)

Six groups of $PG_1$, from A to F are classified on the basis of substitutents on the pentane ring.

There are four other types of compound all shown below:

1. PG endoperoxides (PGG and PGH)
2. Thromboxanes (Tx) derived from (1). These are not classical PGs because they do not have the pentane ring
3. Prostacyclin ($PGI_2$)
4. Leukotrienes — made through an alternative non-prostaglandin pathway for AA metabolism

### The arachidonic acid cascade

PGs are derived from essential fatty acids (EFAs) of the linoleic acid family.

The major (possibly sole) role of EFAs is to supply a precursor pool for PG synthesis.

The minimum linoleic acid requirements in the diet of adults is 5 per cent of calorific intake.

DGLA and AA circulate as their esters. The action of a lipase to produce free acids is therefore necessary before the major enzyme

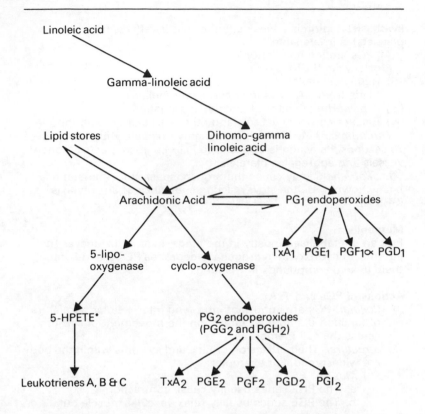

Linoleic acid

Gamma-linoleic acid

Lipid stores                    Dihomo-gamma
                                linoleic acid

            Arachidonic Acid ⇄ PG₁ endoperoxides

5-lipo-                              TxA₁  PGE₁  PGF₁α  PGD₁
oxygenase      cyclo-oxygenase

5-HPETE*            PG₂ endoperoxides
                   (PGG₂ and PGH₂)

Leukotrienes A, B & C    TxA₂  PGE₂  PGF₂  PGD₂  PGI₂

* 5-hydroxyperoxy arachidonic (or eicosatetraenoic) acid

*cyclo-oxygenase* can act. This is probably a major rate limiting step in PG biosynthesis. Several hormones, drugs and other substances affect PG synthesis by inhibiting release of AA, e.g.

(i)  TSH activates phospholipase to stimulate PG synthesis in the thyroid

(ii) Glucocorticoids block phosphatase to inhibit PG synthesis.

*PG cyclo-oxygenase* (or synthetase) is a glycoprotein (MW 126 000) with polypeptide, haem and carbohydrate moieties.

It can be inhibited irreversibly by fatty acids in high concentrations.

Non-steroidal anti-inflammatory drugs (NSAID) also inhibit it. Indomethacin has a potent but temporary effect. Fenamates are also potent but their value is limited by the side-effects produced due to their ability to antagonise PG actions as well as inhibit synthesis. Aspirin is a weak inhibitor but its effects (e.g. on platelets) is irreversible.

All PGs are interconvertable.

Prostacyclin (PGI$_2$) is
 (i) Highly unstable
 (ii) Made from AA by blood vessel endothelium
 (iii) A powerful inhibitor of platelet aggregation
 (iv) Relaxes coronary vessels and other vascular smooth muscle

Thromboxane A$_2$ (TxA$_2$) is also highly unstable with a half life of 30 seconds. Its action is opposite to PGI$_2$ i.e. it contracts coronary vessels and aggregates platelets.

Leukotriene C may cause the bronchospasm of asthma. It has been shown to be the slow reacting substance of anaphylaxis (SRS-A).

## Metabolism
PGs are metabolised mostly in the lungs, liver and kidneys. The enzyme 15-hydroxy-dehydrogenase degrades PGs E and F into their 15-keto compounds in the lungs.

## Actions of PGs and TxA$_2$
1. *Cellular.* PGs are important intra- and inter-cellular regulators of function due to their effects on the movement of calcium across the cell membrane.
2. *Structural.* Their effects on organs and systems within the body are widespread. For example:
    (i) *Muscle*
        a. The PGF series usually cause contraction
        b. The PGE series usually relax vascular muscle but contract gut muscle
        c. PGI$_2$ relaxes and TxA$_2$ constricts vascular muscle
    e.g. PGF$_{2a}$ constricts the ductus arteriosus and the PGEs and PGI$_2$ dilate it.
    (ii) *Platelets*
        a. PG endoperoxides and TxA$_2$ induce platelet aggregation and activation
        b. PGE$_1$, high concentrations of PGE$_2$, PGD$_2$ and prostacyclin inhibit this reaction strongly
    (iii) *Immune system*
        PGs act as 'fine-tuners' of immune function. They are involved in the maturation and function of T lymphocytes; they help to control B lymphocytes and suppressor T cells; and they regulate lymphokine secretion
    (iv) *Uterus*
        a. Progesterone enhances the capacity of oestrogen to stimulate PG synthesis and together they alter the PGF/PGE production ratio

b. The highest concentration of PGF$_{2a}$ in the endometrium occurs during the mid-to-late luteal phase; PGE has no cyclical variation. The significance of this is unclear. It could account for the cyclical alteration in the pattern of myometrial activity and vasoconstriction of spiral arterioles producing menstruation

c. The action of PGF on myometrium alters in pregnancy. In the non-pregnant uterus PGF contracts myometrium and PGE relaxes it.
In pregnancy both PGE$_2$ and PGF$_{2a}$ contract myometrium

d. PGs may initiate labour but the evidence is only circumstantial.

e. PGs facilitate the action of oxytocin and are released during oxytocin-induced contractions. The uterine response to oxytocin and the degree of PG release are increased by oestrogen

f. The decidua, fetal membranes and placenta can synthesise PGs but their concentration in decidua is low (due to suppression by the conceptus?)

g. PGs may help to regulate utero-placental blood flow

h. They may also be involved in the changes which occur in collagen as pregnancy advances. These changes cause 'cervical ripening' and may lead to rupture of the membranes

FURTHER READING

Horrotin, D. F. (1978) *Prostaglandins: Physiology, Pharmacology and Clinical Significance.* Edinburgh: Churchill Livingstone.
Oliver, T. K. & Kirschbaum, T. H. (1980) Seminars in Perinatology. Prostaglandin Symposium, Vol IV, Nos. 1 and 2. New York: Grune and Stratton.

## SEXUAL RESPONSES

Masters and Johnson described sexual responses in men and women as having four phases given the acronym EPOR.

*Excitement phase*. Psychogenic and physical stimuli cause sexual arousal. During this and the next phase genital vasocongestion occurs producing penile erection in the male and vaginal congestion and lubrication in the female.
The phase can last for minutes or hours.

*Plateau phase*. The arousal and tension becomes generally manifest. In women a skin flush appears and carpopedal spasm may occur. It lasts for seconds or minutes. If stimuli are inadequate the response does not proceed and the arousal subsides slowly.

*Orgasmic phase.* Reflex, clonic striated and smooth muscle contractions occur for a few seconds. This is most manifest as ejaculation in the male and uterovaginal contractions in the female. Sexual tension is relieved in a climax of intense pleasure. It has no obvious physical purpose but rather helps to bind the partners together psychologically and spiritually.

*Resolution phase.* The pelvic haemodynamics return to normal. It lasts for some minutes or hours if orgasm has not occurred.

In the male an *absolute refractory period* follows during which it is not possible to arouse him by renewed sexual stimulation. Its length depends on age (the older the man the longer it lasts) and psychological factors e.g. the erotic stimulus. There is no such refractory period in women.

**The role of sex steroids**
Androgens are necessary for male sexuality in that they stimulate sexual appetite (libido) and maintain ejaculatory mechanism (but not erection).

In women the effect of oestrogen on libido and arousability is uncertain. They may act in concert with androgens which also play a role in stimulating sexual appetite in the female. The effect of progesterone may vary depending on its ratio with oestrogen.

FURTHER READING

Elstein, M. (ed.) (1980) Sexual Medicine. *Clinics in Obstetrics and Gynaecology*, Vol. 7, No. 2. London: W. B. Saunders
Masters, W. H. & Johnson, V. E. (1966) *Human Sexual Responses.* Boston: Little, Brown

# Developmental biology

## THE PLACENTA

The placenta is an organ of fetal and maternal origin, the main function of which is the exchange of nutrients and waste products.
The human placenta is:
1. *Chorio-allantoic* — it is vascularised by vessels homologous with the allantoic vessels of lower mammals
2. *Haemochorial* — only trophoblast, connective tissue and fetal endothelium intervene between maternal and fetal circulation
3. *Villous*
4. *Deciduate* — maternal decidua are shed at and after birth
5. *Discoidal*

### Morphology of the placenta
1. The *umbilical cord* contains one vein and two arteries. The umbilical vein terminates within the fetal abdomen when it joins with the ductus venosus. It contains the most highly oxygenated blood which also carries the highest concentration of nutrients.
      The umbilical arteries are the main continuation of the fetal internal iliac arteries and carry de-oxygenated blood to the placenta
2. *Cotyledons* develop by progressive branching of the primary vascular trunk and the formation of villi. There are about 200 of varying size in each placenta each containing a single spiral artery and vein separated from the intervillous space by trophoblast
3. *Lobes* are formed by the grouping together and Interdigitation of cotyledons. There are usually between 20 and 40 lobes giving the characteristic appearance of the maternal surface of the placenta. There is no vascular anastomosis within or between cotyledons

### Important features of the placenta
1. It grows throughout pregnancy; new villi are formed up to term and there is capacity for compensating hypertrophy

2. Despite the fact that up to 30 per cent of villi can often be rendered functionless by perivillous fibrin deposition, the fetus is not compromised. There must therefore be a large functional reserve.
   (Note: this fibrin deposition is not to be confused with infarction which does compromise the fetus and is associated with widespread maternal arteriolar thrombosis)
3. The mechanism by which maternal blood flow to the placenta is controlled is unknown. The spiral arterioles which open directly into the intervillous space cannot do so because their muscular wall is destroyed and replaced by trophoblast
4. Placental weight is a poor indicator of its functional adequacy. Fetal growth is not determined by placental size. The small placenta is a manifestation not a cause of poor fetal growth
   The correlation between the weights of the placenta and fetus are not particularly strong (correlation coefficient 0.5–0.6) suggesting that the placenta has some capacity for independent growth.

## Protein hormones of the placenta

*1. Human chorionic gonadotrophin (hCG)*
 (i) hCG is a glycoprotein which differs from LH only by the 28–30 terminal amino acids of its beta-subunit
 (ii) Its half life is 24 hours
(iii) It is secreted by syncytiotrophoblast
(iv) It is measurable in the circulation within 8 days of conception
 (v) It maintains corpus luteum function for the first 10 weeks of pregnancy.
      It may also stimulate steroidogenesis in the early fetal testes and the inner zone of the fetal adrenal
(iv) It has a weak thyrotrophic action

*2. Human chorionic thyrotrophin (hCT)*
 (i) hCT is present in very small amounts in the normal placenta
(ii) In molar pregnancy it may have significant effects on the thyroid gland

*3. Human chorionic adreno-cortical trophic hormone (hCACTH)*
Cortisol levels in pregnant women are resistant to suppression by dexamethasone suggesting the presence of an autonomous placental ACTH.

*4. Human placental lactogen (hPL)*
  (i) hPL is a single chain polypeptide held together by two disulphide bonds
 (ii) Chemically it is 90 per cent similar to growth hormone but it has only 3 per cent of its activity
(iii) Its half life is about 30 minutes

(iv) It is produced by syncytiotrophoblast
(v) Its metabolic role is to mobilise lipids as free fatty acids thus providing the fetus with a constant energy source
(vi) It antagonises the peripheral action of insulin
(vii) Maternal levels of hPL correlate with fetal and placental weight
(viii) The mean level at 35 to 38 weeks' gestation is between 5 and 6 mg/ml

**Other placental proteins**
The syncytiotrophoblast produces a large number of proteins. Among them are:
(i) *SP₁* — β₁ specific glycoprotein, the function of which is unknown
(ii) *PAPP-A and B* — Pregnancy-associated plasma proteins A and B are glycoproteins. PAPP-A is an α₂ macroglobulin which is a potent inhibitor of fibrinolysis. PAPP-B is a β₁ globulin but its function is unknown
(iii) *PP5* is a glycoprotein which inhibits protease. Its function is unknown but it is elevated in pre-eclampsia

**THE FETO-PLACENTAL UNIT**
The fetus and placenta grow and function as one unit, e.g. in the production of steroid hormones. Separately they lack some vital enzymes but they function together in steroidogenesis drawing on maternal resources and relying on her for clearance.

*Steroid hormone production*
The charts below show the main pathways and enzyme blocks in steroid production by the feto-placental unit.
1. *Progesterone* is largely produced by the corpus luteum until about 10 weeks' gestation after which the placenta takes over. The corpus luteum is vital for continuation of the pregnancy until about the seventh week.

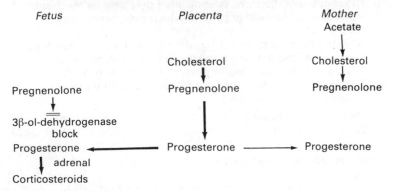

**Production of progesterone**
The most important role for progesterone in pregnancy is to
provide a substrate pool for the fetal adrenal to produce gluco- and
mineralocorticosteroids.
   It is also catabolic. The sodium balance in pregnancy is partly
due to a balance of actions between aldosterone (sodium sparing)
and progesterone (sodium losing).
   2. *Oestrogens* are produced from androgens which come from
      the maternal blood stream in early pregnancy. By
      mid-pregnancy the substrate is predominantly (90 per cent)
      dehydroepiandrosterone sulphate (DHA sulphate) from the
      fetal adrenal.
   The first pathway illustrated is for oestrone and oestradiol.

**Production of oestrogens** (See page 57)
   During pregnancy oestrone and oestradiol excretion increases by
a factor of 100 compared to the non-pregnant state but oestriol
excretion increases by a factor of 1000. The functions of oestrogen
in pregnancy are ill-defined. They stimulate growth of the uterus
and breast and probably have important fetal effects.
   The *fetal adrenal gland* is differentiated by seven weeks'
gestation into a thick inner fetal and thus outer cortical zone. By the
end of the third trimester it is larger than the fetal kidney but it
slowly decreases in size thereafter only to begin a second growth
phase at about 34 weeks' gestation.
   The fetal zone's primary function may be to provide DHA sulphate
for oestriol synthesis under the control of hCG.

**THE FETUS**

**1. Fetal growth**
  (i) The total number of cells in a term fetus arise by 42 successive
      divisions of the fertilised ovum
 (ii) A mere five further cell divisions suffice to attain adult size
(iii) The number of divisions is controlled precisely by mechanisms
      (such as modification enzymes) which programme cell
      differentiation
 (iv) Growth hormone does not regulate growth directly but does so
      through second messengers such as the *somatomedins*.
      Thyroid hormone is also important for proper growth
  (v) The average weight of normal fetuses as pregnancy
      progresses are as follows

| Menstrual age (weeks) | 10 : | 20 : | 30 : | 40 |
|---|---|---|---|---|
| Weight (g) about | 5 : | 300 : | 1500 : | 3420 |

**2. Factors affecting fetal growth**
Among these are:
  (i) *Genetic control.* This predominates in the first half of

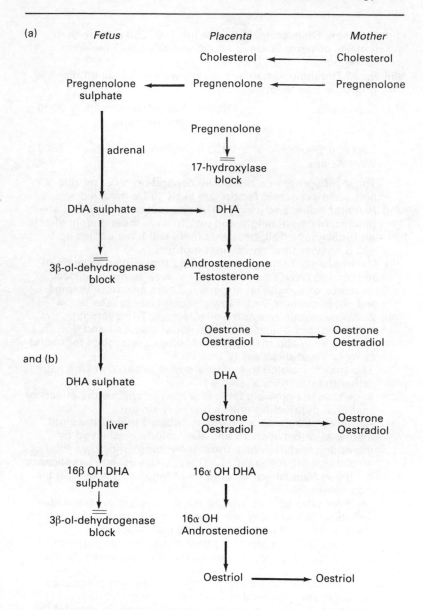

pregnancy but environmental factors and other constraints give rise to greater variability in the second half of pregnancy. About 15 per cent of total birthweight variation is attributable to the fetal genotype

(ii) *Fetal sex.* On average males weigh 150–200 g more than females at term. There is no difference up to 33 weeks' gestation

(iii) *Race.* The approximate mean birthweight for six ethnic groups are as follows:

| Europeans | 3200 g | Indonesians and Africans | 3000 g |
|---|---|---|---|
| East and South West Asians | 3100 g | Indians | 2900 g |

These differences do not solely depend on race; nutritional and socio-economic factors are likely to be involved

(iv) *Parental height and weight.* The paternal contribution is solely genetic. Maternal height and weight have independent effects on birthweight. Tall, heavy mothers will have babies up to 500 g heavier than short, light mothers

(i) *Maternal age.* Teenage mothers and those over 35 years of age tend to have smaller babies (as well as an increased incidence of congenital anomaly). There are more younger and older mothers in the lower social classes (see below)

(vi) *Socio-economic and nutritional factors.* The average birthweight of babies born into social classes I and II (professional and managerial) is 150 g greater than for babies born into social classes IV and V

This may be related to maternal size, age and smoking habits rather than nutritional status

In general the growing fetus is protected against the effects of maternal deprivation unless it is very severe

A study in Guatemala, however, showed that birthweight increases of between 28 and 80 g could be achieved by increasing dietary intake throughout pregnancy by a total of 10 000 kcal (42 megajoules). This may be of little significance for the individual but it could be of long-term benefit in the population

Mothers who gain no weight during pregnancy have babies weighing 300 to 400 g less than those who gain 20 kg or more

(vii) *Birth order.* Birthweight rises from first to second pregnancies by about 130 g with a smaller rise in the third pregnancy. This may be associated with increased maternal weight

(viii) *Previous obstetric history.* Women whose first pregnancy ended in stillbirth tend to have relatively small babies in subsequent pregnancies. No such effect can be noted if the first pregnancy ended in spontaneous abortion

(ix) *Smoking and altitude.* Smoking in pregnancy reduces the mean birthweight by 100 to 200 g from 34 weeks' gestation onwards. Nicotine and carbon monoxide pass through the placenta readily

Birthweight falls by about 100 g for every 1000 metres of altitude

3. **Weight for gestation standards**
   (i) Weight for gestation standards are statistical reference levels which enable babies from similar populations to be defined and compared in a uniform manner in terms of weight and gestational age
   (ii) Standard percentile values for birthweight can be found in tabular form in *Diagnostic Indices in Pregnancy* by F. E. Hytten and T. Lind. Documenta Geigy, 1972, p. 84 and in nomogram form in the *British Journal of Obstetrics and Gynaecology*, 87, 2, p. 81, 1980
   (iii) Size (as assessed by weight) at birth is important because statistically, when the prognosis for an infant is dependent on the two variables, birthweight and gestational age, birthweight proves to be the more important
   (iv) Most of the infants in whom problems will arise are found in the group found weighing less than the tenth percentile for gestation. These infants are termed 'small-for-dates' (SFD) or 'light-for-dates' (LFD), 'or small-for-gestational age' (SGA)
   (v) The common standard selects a higher proportion of female than male infants from first rather than subsequent pregnancies because the average female infant is lighter than the average male and first babies tend to be lighter than subsequent ones
   (vi) Corrections are therefore made for gestational age and sex and can be made for birth order
   (vii) The tenth percentile cut-off for gestational age and sex for defining SFD infants is useful in clinical practice. Lowering the percentiles to the fifth or the third is useful in clinical research
   (viii) The clinical prediction that an infant will be born SFD is surprisingly poor as is shown below

| | Detection rate |
|---|---|
| Infants under the tenth percentile | 30% |
| Infants under the fifth percentile | 50% |
| Infants under the third percentile | 70% |

4. **Factors associated with intrauterine growth retardation** (infants under the tenth percentile for gestational age and sex).
   (i) Maternal height — an excess of short mothers (1.50 m or less)
   (ii) Maternal weight — an excess of light mothers
   (iii) Smoking
   (iv) Low social class (NB in social classes IV and V 50 per cent smoke: In social class I 15 per cent smoke).

(v) Chronic hypertension
(vi) Moderate to severe pre-eclampsia
(vii) Previous stillbirth
(viii) Previous SFD liveborn sibling
(ix) Mother herself SFD

5. **Factors associated with large-for-dates infants** (greater than the 90th percentile for gestational age and sex).
(i) Height — tall mothers
(ii) Weight for height ratio
(iii) Good weight gain
(ix) Second to fourth pregnancies
(v) Maternal age 20 to 30 years
(vi) Smoking deficit
(vii) Previous large for dates sibling
(viii) High maternal and/or paternal birthweight

6. **Assessment of fetal growth**
(i) *Height of uterine fundus*
Clinical judgement of fundal height is not an accurate measure of gestational age but gives a guide to fetal growth. It is best measured as height (cm) above symphysis pubis as follows:

| Gestational age (weeks) | Average height (cm) | + 2 SDs |
|---|---|---|
| 20–31 | Height = weeks | ± 3 |
| 32–36 | Height = (weeks — 1) | ± 3 |
| 37–38 | Height = (weeks — 2) | ± 3 |
| 39–40 | Height = (weeks — 3) | ± 3 |

(ii) *Ultrasound — crown-rump (C-R) length*
At 7 weeks menstrual age the C-R length is 10 mm. This has increased to 55 mm by 12 weeks. (It provides an accurate estimate of gestational age up to 14 weeks)
(iii) *Ultrasound — cephalometry*
Apart from clinical assessment this is the most widely used measured of fetal growth (see below)
When used to indicate fetal maturity it is most accurate before 24 weeks, but unreliable after 34 weeks' gestation
(iv) *Ultrasound — head abdomen ratio*
Ultrasonic measurement of the ratio of the head circumference (at the level of the third ventricle) and the abdominal circumference (at the level of the umbilical vein) is a useful measure of fetal growth
It is especially useful in suspected intrauterine growth retardation (IUGR) when sparing of head growth makes BPD measurement less reliable

| Head: Abdomen Ratio | Gestational age (weeks) | Approx. mean BPD (cm) | Increase (per 4 wks) (cm) |
|---|---|---|---|
| 1.2 | 16 | 3.5 ⎤ |  |
| 1.2 | 20 | 5.0 ⎬ | 1.5 |
| 1.15 | 24 | 6.5 ⎦ |  |
| 1.1 | 28 | 7.5 ⎤ |  |
| 1.05 to 1.0 | 32 | 8.5 ⎬ | 1.0 |
| 1.0 | 36 | 9.5 ⎦ |  |
| 0.95 | 40 | 10.0 | 0.5 |

(v) *Ossification centres*
Radiology will reveal calcification of fetal epiphyses but their appearance is delayed in IUGR

|  | *Average time of appearance* |
|---|---|
| Os calcis | 24 to 26 weeks |
| Distal femoral epiphysis ⎤ | 36 weeks |
| Proximal tubal epiphysis ⎬ |  |
| Femoral head ⎦ | 40 weeks |

## 7. Fetal circulation
   (i) Oxygenated blood (65–80 per cent $O_2$ saturation) passes in the *umbilical vein* to the liver
  (ii) Most of it travels in the ductus venosus to the *inferior vena cava* (*IVC*). The remainder supplies the left two-thirds of the liver by offshoots of the umbilical vein (the right one-third receives blood from the portal vein) and then passes to the IVC via the *hepatic veins*
 (iii) The IVC adds de-oxygenated blood from the abdomen, pelvis and lower limbs
 (iv) Blood entering the *right atrium* from the IVC is directed through the *foramen ovale* to the left atrium
  (v) Blood from the *superior vena cava* (*SVC*) passes through the right atrium to the right ventricle. There are therefore cross-streams of blood in the right atrium but there is some intermingling
 (vi) From the left atrium blood (60 per cent $O_2$ saturation) passes to the *left ventricle* and then the ascending *aorta*
(vii) It supplies the head, neck and upper limbs and returns via jugular and subclavian veins to the SVC (see 'v)
(viii) From the right atrium and ventricle it is pumped into the *pulmonary trunk*
 (ix) Most of it enters the *ductus arteriosus* which is wide and lies in the line of flow
  (x) A small quantity circulates through the lungs to return to the left atrium by the pulmonary veins

(xi)  Blood from the ductus arteriosus is deflected into the descending aorta

(xii)  Most of this returns to the placenta in the *umbilical arteries:* the residue supplies the trunk and lower limbs

FURTHER READING

Hytten, F. E. & Chamberlain, C. V. P. (1980) *Clinical Physiology in Obstetrics*. Oxford: Blackwell

Quilligan, E. J. & Kretchmer N. (1980 *Fetal and Maternal Medicine*. Chichester: John Wiley & Sons.

Speroff, L., Glass, R. H. & Kase, N. G. (1978) *Clinical Gynecologic Endocrinology and Infertility*, 2nd edn. Baltimore: Williams and Wilkins

# Maternal accommodation in pregnancy

## CARDIOVASCULAR SYSTEM

1. *Plasma volume*
   - (i) It increases progressively to its maximum at 34 weeks
   - (ii) The mean increase $\begin{cases} \text{in primigravidae is about 1250 ml} \\ \text{in multigravidae is about 1500 ml} \end{cases}$
   - (iii) From 34 weeks the volume falls by 200 to 300 ml
   - (iv) A further drop of 500 to 600 ml occurs at delivery
   - (v) It has returned to non-pregnant levels by six to eight weeks postpartum
2. *Cardiac output*
   - (i) It rises by about 1.5 litres/minute within the first 10 weeks of pregnancy and is maintained at this level
3. The *sleeping heart rate* is raised by about 15 beats/minute. Ectopic beats are common and episodes of supra-ventricular tachycardia may occur
4. The *stroke volume rises* from 64 ml to 71 ml from early pregnancy
5. The *arterio-venous oxygen difference* of the blood is reduced because cardiac output is raised with a smaller rise in oxygen consumption. It is at its lowest in early pregnancy
6. *Blood pressure*
   - (i) The *systolic blood pressure* (SBP) falls slightly in early pregnancy but rises again in late pregnancy
   - (ii) The *diastolic blood pressure* (DBP) is well below non-pregnant levels from early in pregnancy. It returns to those levels after 30 to 32 weeks' gestation
   - (iii) The *pulse pressure* is therefore increased in the first and second trimesters
   - (iv) Blood pressure falls significantly during sleep
   - (v) Uterine contractions in labour are associated with a rise in blood pressure
7. *Peripheral resistance* is low at the beginning of pregnancy but gradually increases thereafter
8. *Circulation time* changes very little
9. *Venous pressure* is greatly increased in the femoral and other

leg veins but not in the arms. This is due to compression of the inferior vena cava by uterus and fetus, and the pressure of blood returning from the uterus. About 300 ml of blood is expelled from the uterus during a contraction
10. *Position of the heart*. The *heart* increases in size and it is pushed upwards and forwards. This may produce the following ECG changes
    (i) T wave flattening or reversal in lead III
    (ii) Depression of S-T segment in both chest and limb leads (possibly)
    (iii) Lower voltage QRS complexes
    (iv) Deep Q waves and occasional U waves

## RESPIRATORY SYSTEM

**1. Anatomical changes**
  (i) The lower ribs flare out; the subcostal angle increases from 68° in early pregnancy to 103° at term
 (ii) The transverse diameter of the chest increases by 2 cm
(iii) The diaphragm is raised 4 cm and its excursion in breathing is greater

**2. Respiratory function**
   (i) The *respiratory rate* does not change
  (ii) The *tidal volume* (the volume of gas inspired and expired in each respiration) rises progressively in pregnancy by 0.1 to 0.2 litres
 (iii) The *expiratory reserve* volume (the maximum amount of air expired from the resting end-expiratory positions) falls by about 200 ml (15 per cent)
 (iv) The *residual volume* (the volume of gas remaining at the end of maximal expiration excluding that in dead space) falls by 20 per cent from about 1500 ml to 1200 ml. This fall, combined with the increased tidal volume, causes more efficient gas mixing
  (v) *Vital capacity* (the maximum volume of gas which can be expired after maximum inspiration) may increase by 100 to 100 ml from mid-pregnancy in some women
 (vi) *Inspiratory capacity* (the maximum volume of gas which can be inspired from the resting end expiratory position) rises by about 300 ml (5 per cent)
(vii) The *minute volume* (tidal volume × respiration rate) increases by 40 per cent
(viii) *Airway resistance* is reduced possibly by an increase in airway cross-section

**3. Gas exchange**
  (i) *Oxygen consumption* rises by about 32 ml/min (i.e. 15 per

cent) in late pregnancy. This rise is coped with by the increased oxygen-carrying capacity of the blood

(ii) The increase in ventilation in pregnancy greatly exceeds the increase in oxygen consumption. The alveolar concentration of $CO_2$, therefore, falls

(iii) *Alveolar $P_{CO_2}$* falls slightly in the luteal phase of the cycle and this fall continues in pregnancy. This may be a progesterone effect

(iv) The respiratory centres are more sensitive to changes in $P_{CO_2}$ possibly due to oestrogens. For every 1 mmHg rise in $P_{CO_2}$ in the non-pregnant ventilation increases by 1.5 l/min. In pregnancy the increase is 6 l/min. This may cause some dyspnoea and reduces maternal plasma bicarbonate and thus plasma sodium and osmolality. The fetus benefits by being able to get rid of $CO_2$ without itself having a high $P_{CO_2}$

## THE HAEMATOLOGICAL SYSTEM

### Red cells

1. In women not given iron supplements the increase in *red cell mass* is about 240 ml (18 per cent). For those given iron it is about 400 ml (30 per cent). The increase is linear from the end of the first trimester to term and is probably due to a rise in erythropoietin levels. This increase is proportionately less than the increase in plasma volume. The concentration of red cells in the blood therefore falls

2. The *haematocrit* falls also from about 0.40 to 0.31 in healthy women not taking iron supplements. The reduction is modified by iron

3. The mean minimum *haemoglobin* concentration is 11 to 12 g/dl found at about 34 weeks gestation. There is slight reactivation of HbF production during pregnancy which is an hCG effect

4. The *MCHC* (mean corpuscular haemoglobin concentration) changes very little. The MCV is a more helpful index

5. There is no real change in *MCV* (mean cell volume) but a fall is the earliest effect of iron deficiency

6. *Red cell fragility* increases. They are more spherical due to a fall in colloid osmotic pressure, and are therefore more susceptible to rupture when they take up water

### White cells

The total white cell count (WCC) rises in pregnancy which is almost totally due to an increase in neutrophil polymorphonuclear leucocytes. Mean total WCC is around $9.0 \times 10^9$/l.

1. *Neutrophils* reach their peak level at 30 weeks and plateau thereafter. The mean total WCC is around $6.6 \times 10^9$/l. There is a further neutrophil leucocytosis at the onset of labour but levels

have returned to non-pregnant levels by six days postpartum
2. *Eosinophils* are markedly reduced in number during labour and are virtually absent at delivery. They have risen to non-pregnant levels by the third postpartum day
3. The *lymphocyte* count alters little and there is no consistent change in the number of circulating T and B cells (for function see Immune system — p. 43)

**Platelets**
The platelet count decreases slightly (see Coagulation system — p. 68).

**Iron metabolism**
1. *Iron requirements* in the second and third trimesters are about 2.7 mg/day to allow for fetal needs and blood loss at delivery. Lactation adds another 0.8 mg/day to the requirements
2. The normal daily diet contains 10 to 15 mg of iron of which only five to ten per cent is absorbed. Of that 65 per cent is used in haemoglobin synthesis
3. *Serum iron concentration* is reduced by one-third in late pregnancy. This is modified but not prevented by iron supplements
4. *Iron-binding capacity* doubles during pregnancy
5. *Ferritin* decreases rapidly in early pregnancy. This implies reduction in iron stores but these do not reach 'iron deficiency' levels if iron supplements are given

**Are iron supplements necessary?**
Even with maximum amounts of iron in her diet, the pregnant woman cannot cover the increased demands by increased absorption. Her iron stores must therefore fall. This would suggest that supplementation is necessary. However, there is no convincing clinical evidence that it is routinely worthwhile.

**Folate metabolism**
1. Folate is essential to cell growth and division because it supplies single-carbon fragments to the synthetic pathways. The more active the tissue the more dependent it is on folate coenzymes
   In pregnancy requirements of folate are raised
   (i) To meet the needs of the growing fetus and placenta
   (ii) Because of uterine hypertrophy
   (iii) Because of expanded maternal red cell mass
2. Folate is obtained from fresh green vegetables, liver and kidney as folic acid which is reduced at a cellular level to dihydrofolic then tetrahydrofolic acids
3. The placenta transports folate actively to the fetus in the face of any maternal deficiency

4. The pregnant woman requires a folate intake of 1.8 mmol (or 800 μg) per day to meet all the requirements
5. Plasma folate falls as pregnancy advances reaching half of its non-pregnant value by term
6. Red cell folate makes up 95 per cent of blood folate and is a more useful measure of folate status than plasma folate because it is not subject to such variations
    (i) There is a slight downward trend in red cell folate levels in pregnancy
    (ii) Levels of <180 nmol/l (<80 ng/ml) are often associated with megaloblastic anaemia
    (iii) Red cell folate levels can be maintained by 100 μg supplements of folic acid daily
    (iv) Although chronic folate deficiency has been linked with miscarriage, fetal anomaly, preterm labour and placental abruption, there is no convincing evidence that a policy of routine folate supplementation during pregnancy has affected their incidence. However, the number of cases of megaloblastic anaemia has been reduced markedly, and in areas of chronic under-nutrition, increases in birthweight have been noted

**Vitamin B12**

Vitamin B12 levels fall in pregnancy being at their lowest
  (i) at 16 to 20 weeks
  (ii) in multiple pregnancy
  (iii) in smokers
   Vitamin B12 deficiency causing pernicious anaemia is rare in the reproductive years and is usually associated with infertility. It may occur during pregnancy associated with chronic folate deficiency
  (i) In women with chronic tropical sprue
  (ii) In strict vegans who eat no food derived from animals

**COAGULATION SYSTEM AND FIBRINOLYSIS**

When small blood vessels are damaged the problem is dealt with predominantly by *platelets* which
 1. Adhere to the damaged vessel wall and bridge any defect
 2. Become activated to release ADP, serotonin, catecholamines, platelet factor 4, and lysosomal enzymes among other vaso-active substances. They also change shape and develop pseudopodia by which they link together
 3. Stimulate further platelet aggregation

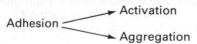

4. The coagulation cascade is triggered
In large vessel damage activation of the coagulation cascade and vasoconstriction are the predominant responses.

## Coagulation factors

| Factor | Alternative name |
| --- | --- |
| I | Fibrinogen |
| II | Prothrombin |
| III | Tissue thromboplastin |
| IV | Calcium ions (Ca++) |
| V | Proaccelerin |
| (No factor VI) | |
| VII | Factor VII |
| VIII | Antihaemophilic Factor |
| IX | Christmas Factor |
| X | Stuart-Prower Factor |
| XI | Plasma thromboplastin antecedent |
| XII | Hagemann Factor |
| XIII | Fibrin-stabilising Factor |

Although these factors are only present in picogram quantities a sequential series of enzyme conversions in the coagulation cascade lead to the conversion of milligrams of fibrinogen to fibrin. Biochemical amplification is therefore by a mathematical factor of $10^9$.

## Blood coagulation

*The coagulation cascade*

This has a preliminary phase followed by three distinct phases.
    *Preliminary phase.* During this the coagulation cascade generates enough energy to convert prothrombin to thrombin (Phase 1).

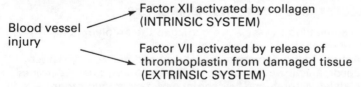

Blood vessel injury
→ Factor XII activated by collagen (INTRINSIC SYSTEM)
→ Factor VII activated by release of thromboplastin from damaged tissue (EXTRINSIC SYSTEM)

The intrinsic system is relatively slow, taking between five and 20 minutes to produce visible fibrin. The extrinsic (or tissue factor) system accelerates the process forming fibrin within 12 seconds.
    *Phase 1.* The intrinsic and extrinsic systems follow a common pathway following activation of Factor X. Aided by Factor V prothrombin is converted to thrombin which acts as a proteolytic enzyme.

## COAGULATION
### The coagulation cascade

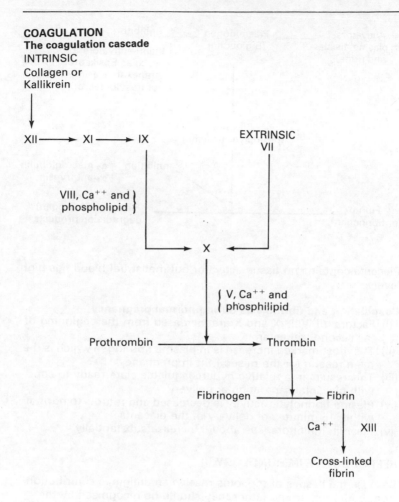

INTRINSIC
Collagen or
Kallikrein

XII ⟶ XI ⟶ IX

EXTRINSIC
VII

VIII, $Ca^{++}$ and
phospholipid

X

V, $Ca^{++}$ and
phosphilipid

Prothrombin ⟶ Thrombin

Fibrinogen ⟶ Fibrin

$Ca^{++}$ | XIII

Cross-linked
fibrin

*Phase 2* involves the production of stable fibrin from fibrinogen. Fibrinogen is made up of three pairs of polypeptide chains linked by disulphide bonds. Two pairs of small peptides (fibrinopeptide A & B) are split off by thrombin to produce monomeric fibrin which then polymerises. Factor XIII stabilises the fibrin.

*Phase 3* is the gradual process of fibrin retraction during wound healing.

### Fibrinolysis
The components of the fibrinolytic system are shown below.

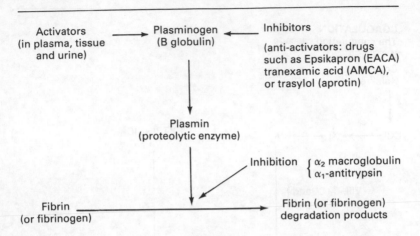

Placenta contains no tissue activator but menstrual blood has high levels.

### Coagulation and fibrinolysis during normal pregnancy
  (i) Factors VII, VIII, IX and X are increased from the beginning of the second trimester
 (ii) The most marked increase is in plasma fibrinogen which is the main reason for the raised ESR in pregnancy
(iii) This results in a relative hypercoagulable state ready to cope with placental separation at delivery
 (iv) Plasma fibrinolytic activity is decreased and returns to normal within 15 minutes of delivery of the placenta
  (v) Plasmin inhibitors (see above) increase substantially

### REPRODUCTIVE IMMUNOLOGY
Because the tissues of the fetus receive an antigenic contribution from both mother and father they should be recognised by the maternal immune system as at least being partially 'foreign'.

Analogies with other 'transplants' suggest that it should therefore be rejected. The mechanism by which this is prevented are complex and ill-understood due to limitations in the methods available for their investigation. Our present understanding can be summarised as follows:

### 1. Pre-implantation
  (i) Major histocompatibility antigens are not expressed on the zygote therefore sensitisation and rejection cannot occur
 (ii) The zona pellucida may act to a minor extent as an immune 'quaratining' layer

**2. Post-implantation**
 (i) Maternal decidua lacks lymphatic drainage. This reduces the exposure of tissues at the feto-maternal interface to lymphocytes
 (ii) Non-villous trophoblast expresses HLA antigens and this is possibly the major cause of the anti-HLA antibodies which can be found in at least some pregnancies
 (iii) Villous trophoblast never expresses HLA antigens. Thus, even if lymphocytes become sensitised against paternal HLA antigens on other cells (e.g. non-villous trophoblast) they cannot mount a rejection against villous trophoblast
 (iv) Trophoblast may share non-HLA antigens with lymphocytes and if antibodies are developed to the former this suppresses any potential cytotoxic activity of the latter
 (v) The trophoblast surface membrane is highly negatively charged. This may help repel cytotoxic lymphocytes
 (vi) The placenta acts as a barrier to the passage of maternal (particularly lymphoid) cells to the fetus

**3. Maternal factors**
 (i) Local non-specific immune suppression may occur due to hCG and some pregnancy-specific proteins
 (ii) Specific suppression of immune responses may occur due to immune complexes or suppressor T cells
 (iii) Maternal transferrin binds to the abundant transferrin receptors on the trophoblast surface. This may present an array of maternal antigens at the feto-maternal interface
 These issues are still hotly debated. New techniques (e.g. hybridisation of cells to produce monoclonal antibodies) are likely to advance our understanding considerably.

**URINARY SYSTEM**

*1. Anatomical changes*
 (i) The renal tracts begin to dilate by 10 weeks of pregnancy
 (ii) The changes are usually more marked in the right renal pelvis and ureter
 (iii) The ureteral dilatation terminates at the pelvic brim
 (iv) These changes are partly due to mechanical pressure but not solely. The traditional role of progesterone is now questioned
 (v) There is also hypertrophy of ureteral smooth muscle and the ureters, though dilated, are certainly not toneless
 (vi) Dilatation persists for 12–16 weeks after delivery

*2. Renal haemodynamics*
 (i) Effective renal plasma flow (ERPF) ⎫ increase during
 (ii) Glomerular filtration rate (GFR)  ⎬ pregnancy by
                                        ⎭ 30–50 per cent

The 24 hour creatinine clearance is an indicator of GFR and shows the following features
  (i) Changes begin shortly after conception
 (ii) It rises to between 150 and 200 ml/min by the end of the second trimester
(iii) It tends to fall during the last trimester but this may be artefactual
  Urea and uric acid clearances are also raised causing a fall in their plasma levels.

  3. The filtration fraction increases because the increase in GFR exceeds that of ERPF

**Renal tubular function**
  1. *Uric acid*. Clearance rises and tubular reabsorption falls. Plasma levels therefore fall by about 30 per cent
  2. *Glucose*. Glycosuria is common in pregnant women but its presence and timing are highly variable. It used to be thought that the 'renal threshold' or maximum tubular reabsorptive capacity for glucose (Tm glucose) was frequently exceeded but this concept has been superseded.
     Renal absorption is however, less effective in pregnancy. Glycosuria is not a useful screening test for carbohydrate intolerance in pregnancy
  3. *Amino-acids.* Clearance is increased and up to 2 g amino acids may be lost in the urine each day
  4. *Acid-base balance*. Arterial pH averages 7.44 in pregnant women compared to 7.40 in the non-pregnant. This is due to a loss of hydrogen ions in urine and a mild respiratory alkalosis
  5. *Water*. Plasma osmolality falls within the first eight weeks by about 10 mosm/kg and remains at this reduced level thereafter
     The passage of normal urine volumes in the face of low plasma osmolality and a raised extra-cellular fluid volume is unique to pregnancy. It is due to a re-setting of the osmoreceptors and the maintenance of arginine vasopressin (AVP) secretion
  6. *Potassium.* The potassium sparing action of progesterone prevents its increased urinary loss in the face of relatively alkaline urine, reduced bicarbonate levels, and marked increases in aldosterone and other mineral-corticosteroids
  7. *Sodium*. The increase in tubular reabsorption of sodium is the largest adaptation required of the kidney in pregnancy at a high metabolic cost.
     Sodium is the major solute of the extracellular space and the final pathway of volume control. Among the factors which control sodium excretion are the following

| | |
|---|---|
| GFR increased | Raised aldosterone levels |
| Progesterone | Increase in other potential |
| Naturietic hormones | salt retaining hormones such |
| (e.g. AVP) | as oestrogen, desoxycortico- |
| Decreased plasma albumin | sterone, cortisol, hPl, prolactin |
| Decreased peripheral resistance | Supine and upright position |

**The renin-angiotensin system**
Renin is an enzyme produced in the kidney acting on an α-2
globulin substrate to form an inactive decapeptide *angiotensin I*.
This is converted by another enzyme to *angiotensin II* which
increases blood pressure.
   The changes in pregnancy are:
1. *Plasma renin concentration* rises markedly in the first trimester
   but falls thereafter. Only 10 per cent is active; the rest is
   derived from the myometrium and chorion.
2. *Plasma renin activity* rises two to four-fold within the first
   trimester and remains constant thereafter.
3. *Renin substrate* increases greatly in response to oestrogen,
   particularly in the second half of pregnancy.
4. Plasma *angiotensin II* is markedly elevated although the range
   of values is wide. Normal pregnant women become highly
   resistant to the pressor effects of angiotensin by 10 weeks'
   gestation.

**ENDOCRINE SYSTEM**

**Hypothalamus and pituitary gland**
The activity of the anterior pituitary during pregnancy is modified
greatly by hormones from the fetal-placental unit.

*1. Prolactin*
  (i) Secretion increases throughout pregnancy in response to
      oestrogen stimulation. By term the concentration has
      increased ten to twenty fold.
 (ii) Basal concentrations fall rapidly after delivery but remain
      above the normal range in lactating women.
(iii) Suckling induces a prompt release and levels rise five to ten
      fold.
*Role of prolactin in pregnancy*
  (i) Trophic action on breast and possibly:
 (ii) Maintenance of fetal salt and water balance
(iii) Maintenance of calcium balance through Vitamin D
      metabolism
*Role of prolactin after delivery*
  (i) Initiation and maintenance of lactation

(ii) Prevention of ovulation (and therefore conception) during period of breastfeeding.

2. *Gonadotrophins*
Secretion is inhibited to levels found in the luteal phase of the menstrual cycle. This is a direct effect of the high prolactin levels. Cyclical release of FSH and LH is inhibited during lactation. Follicular development is prevented and oestrogen levels remain low.

3. *Growth hormone*
Secretion is impaired possibly due to the action of hPL.

4. *Corticotrophin*
ACTH levels rise slightly but the source of this rise may be the placenta itself.

5. *Thyrotrophin* (TSH) is unchanged

6. The posterior pituitary hormones *oxytocin* and *vasopressin* are very difficult to measure and the situation in pregnancy is unclear.
Oxytocin levels are low (undetectable in 20 per cent of women). Despite the oxytocin surges associated with labour the physiological function of the hormone during parturition is not clear.

**The adrenal gland**
1. *Aldosterone* levels rise within days of conception due to an increase in angiotensin II. This reaction is necessary in pregnancy to conserve sodium (see p. 73).
2. *Plasma cortisol* levels, both bound and free are elevated with loss of the normal diurnal variation
3. *ll-deoxycorticosterone* (DOC) shows the largest increase of all adrenal steroids starting by eight weeks' gestation. DOC is not suppressible by dexamethasone during pregnancy. It may be intimately involved with parturition (see p. 79)
4. *Plasma testosterone* rises secondary to the rise in sex hormone-binding globulin although it is likely that unbound testosterone is unchanged
5. The catecholamines, adrenaline and noradrenaline, are unchanged during pregnancy

**Thyroid gland**

1. *Iodine*
(i) Renal clearance doubles in the first trimester and then remains stable. It is normal by six weeks postpartum
(ii) The result is a low plasma inorganic iodine

2. *Thyroid hormones*
   (i) Tri-iodothyronine (T₃) is three times more active than thyroxine (T₄)
  (ii) T₃ and T₄ circulate in reverse equilibrium with protein bound hormone. Only 0.5 per cent of T₃ and 0.5 per cent of T₄ are present free in the serum
 (iii) The level of thyroid binding proteins (globulin, pre-albumin and albumin) more than doubles due to an oestrogen effect on the liver
  (iv) The proportion of free T₄ falls and the protein bound iodine (PBI) rises
   (v) This is corrected by an increase in T₄ production
  (vi) Free T₃ and T₄ levels therefore remain unchanged in pregnancy
 (vii) The thyroid also secretes thyrocalcitonin which inhibits bone resorption and therefore lowers serum calcium. Information on pregnancy changes is inadequate
3. *Basal metabolic rate* (BMR) increases by up to 30 per cent by the third trimester. This is necessary because of:
   (i) The requirements of the uterus and fetus (75 per cent of the change)
  (ii) Increased maternal respiratory and cardiac effort (25 per cent of the change)
4. *Thyroid stimulating hormone* (TSH) is probably unchanged in pregnancy
   Chorionic thyrotrophin and long-acting thyroid stimulator (LATS) can affect thyroid function in normal pregnancy.
   LATS is an IgG acting on thyroid microsomes.
   Hydatidiform mole may cause a marked increase in thyroid activity due to molar thyrotrophin.

*Tests of thyroid function in pregnancy*
The *T₃ resin uptake test* (T₃R) and the *free thyroxine index* (FT₄1 = PBI × T₃R) are useful tests of thyroid function in pregnancy because the T₃R is low despite a high PBI (c.f. thyrotoxicosis with high T₃R and PBI).

## CARBOHYDRATE METABOLISM

Normal pregnancy affects glucose homeostasis as follows:
1. Plasma glucose levels fall by about 0.5 mmol during the first trimester and only very slightly thereafter.
2. There is a delay in the time taken to reach peak plasma glucose levels in response to 50 g oral glucose load (37 minutes at 20 weeks' and 55 minutes at 38 weeks' gestation)

3. Basal and post-prandial insulin levels increase by 150 to 300 per cent but this occurs later in pregnancy than the fall in plasma glucose and is not causally related
4. There is tissue resistance to insulin during pregnancy due to
 (i) Reduced cellular uptake of glucose
 (ii) Reduced sensitivity of pancreatic islet & cells (producing glucagon) to insulin
 When blood glucose is being measured a specific enzyme method (e g glucose oxidase) should be used on plasma samples of venous blood.

The British Diabetic Association recommended definition of abnormal carbohydrate tolerance after a 50 g glucose load is:

Venous blood plasma glucose$\geqslant$6.1 mmol/l $\big\}$ at two hours
Capillary blood plasma glucose$\geqslant$6.7 mmol/l

and$\geqslant$8.9 mmol/l $\big\}$ at some other point during the test
 $\geqslant$10.0 mmol/l

## ALIMENTARY FUNCTION AND NUTRITION

### Alimentary function
1. *Appetite* — an early surge occurs which decreases as pregnancy progresses
2. *Daily food intake* — increases by about 1 megajoule (200 kcal) by the beginning of the second trimester
3. *Gastro-intestinal tract*
 (i) Muscle tone and motility are reduced throughout
 (ii) Acid and pepsin secretions fall in the stomach
 (iii) Water reabsorption in the large intestine plus motor sluggishness may lead to constipation
4. *Liver function* — changes very little. Bromsulphthalein (BSP) is cleared more slowly but other tests of function and bilirubin levels are unchanged

*Diet*
1. It is not necessary to supplement the diet of healthy, well-fed pregnant women with protein, minerals or vitamins (except perhaps folic acid)
2. Vitamin D supplements (400 i.u.) daily are indicated in pregnant Asian immigrant women to prevent osteomalacia in the mother and rickets and dental enamel hypoplasia in the fetus
3. The suggested optimum daily calorific intake is 10.0 megajoules (2400 kcal) during pregnancy increasing to 11.5 megajoules (2750 kcal) for lactation

*Calcium metabolism*
The pregnant woman can supply fetal needs while keeping her own skeleton intact. The fall which occurs in calcium is principally due to haemodilution.

*Plasma proteins*
The total protein concentration falls in the first trimester reaching a plateau around mid-pregnancy. This fall is mainly due to reduced albumin concentrations because levels of $\alpha_1$, $\alpha_2$ and $\beta$ globulin fractions rise. The reduction in colloid osmotic pressure parallels that in albumin exactly.
*Serum lipids* rise mainly due to increases in triglycerides. Cholesterol falls initially then increases in a linear fashion to 36 weeks.
Phospholipids also rise.

## WEIGHT GAIN IN PREGNANCY

1. The range of weight gain is wide
2. No single figure can be regarded as 'normal'
3. The optimum is 12.5 kg for the whole of pregnancy and 9 kg for the second half
4. Mothers who gain little or no weight tend to have smaller babies than those who gain more weight
5. One week after delivery the average woman is 4.4 kg above her pre-pregnant weight but this is lost gradually
6. Weight gain in second or subsequent pregnancies is about 1 kg less than during a first pregnancy but this relates to maternal age rather than parity directly
7. Socio-economic status has no influence on weight gain, except in situations of severe malnutrition

### Components of weight gain

| Gestational age | 10 | 20 | 30 | 40 weeks |
|---|---|---|---|---|
| Total maternal weight gain | 650 | 4000 | 8500 | 12500 g |
| Fetus | 5 | 300 | 1500 | 3400 g |
| Placenta | 20 | 170 | 430 | 650 g |
| Amniotic fluid | 30 | 350 | 750 | 800 g |
| Total | 55 | 820 | 2680 | 4850 g |
| Proportion of total maternal weight gain | 8% | 20% | 32% | 40% |

# Parturition

## THE UTERUS DURING PREGNANCY

### 1. Uterine growth
  (i) New muscle is formed only in early pregnancy
 (ii) Hypertrophy is the main feature up to mid-pregnancy and distension thereafter
(iii) Blood vessels grow and become coiled to 20 weeks' gestation and stretch thereafter
 (iv) Uterine weight increases twenty-fold from beginning to end of pregnancy
  (v) Growth is stimulated by mechanical stretching and oestrogens

### 2. Cervical changes before labour
  (i) The cervix softens early in pregnancy due to increased vascularity and gradual replacement of collagen by fluid
 (ii) Slight dilatation can often be noted from about 24 weeks
(iii) Effacement is a late phenomenon

### 3. Uterine activity before labour
  (i) Uterine muscle contracts rhythmically even when isolated; this is regulated by calcium ions
 (ii) As they contract myometrial fibres also retract (i.e. they preserve the same tone but shorten). This is the mechanism by which the physiological lower segment forms late in pregnancy and cervical dilatation occurs during labour
(iii) The myometrium in pregnancy can be stretched greatly without losing the ability to contract and retract maximally (progesterone effect)
 (iv) Progesterone blocks myometrial excitability; sensitivity to oxytocin increases as pregnancy advances; responses to PGs are the same throughout
  (v) Uterine contractions during the first 20 weeks are of high frequency but low intensity
 (vi) Frequency and amplitude increase thereafter
(vii) Irregular, low frequency, high amplitude (Braxton-Hicks) contractions are most apparent in the last two months

(viii) As labour approaches the activity of the fundal myometrium increases most while the lower segment remains relatively inactive. The cervix thus becomes effaced and engagement of the presenting part is encouraged

## INITIATION OF LABOUR

Maternal and feto-placental factors may be involved in the onset of spontaneous labour.

### Maternal factors

1. *Myometrium*
   (i) This remains relatively quiescent despite massive stretching due to the action of progesterone
   (ii) Removal of this block (see below) may facilitate the onset of labour
   (iii) The role of α (stimulatory) and β (inhibitory) adrenergic receptors in initiating labour are uncertain
   (iv) PGs are involved locally in the action of the myometrial cell but are probably not the primary stimulus

2. *Decidua* is a prime source of prostaglandins

3. (i) The *posterior pituitary gland* produces oxytocin but there is no increase in levels before the onset of labour
   (ii) Even during progressive labour it is not clear whether the episodic release of oxytocin is a cause or result of uterine contractions

### Feto-placental factors

1. *The placenta*
   (i) In many animals progesterone levels fall as oestrogens rise near the onset of labour
   (ii) Oestrogen stimulates PG production (see below) and the fall in progesterone increases myometrial excitability
   (iii) Unfortunately the change in the oestrogen/progesterone ratio is much less in humans and no direct relationship between changes and the onset of labour has been shown
   (iv) A facilitatory role for oestrogens in the initiation of labour is suggested by the failure of women to go into labour when there is a placental sulphatase deficiency preventing the synthesis of oestrogens
2. *Fetal membranes*
   The amnion is a potent source of PGs
3. *Fetal pituitary adrenal axis*
   (i) Throughout most of fetal life the main products of the fetal anterior pituitary are the peptide fragments of ACTH

known as α-MSH (α-melanotrophin) and CLIP (corticotrophin-like intermediate lobe peptide) which drive the fetal zone of the adrenal
(ii) A switch occurs to intact ACTH near term which stimulates development of the definitive adrenal cortex
(iii) The production of cortisol by ACTH is important in the initiation of labour in several species (e.g. sheep) but is not essential in Man
(iv) Prolactin is the second trophic agent for the fetal adrenal and it encourages oestrogen production (see p. 31)
4. *Fetal posterior pituitary gland*
Oxytocin is released in the fetus in association with spontaneous labour but it is not known if this is a prime mover or secondary effect

**Possible sequence of events**
1. Progesterone binding protein increases at term: the tissue effects of progesterone decrease
2. The suppression of myometrial excitability by progesterone decreases
3. The relative fall in progesterone also promotes the release of arachidonic acid
4. ACTH promotes DHEA production in the fetal adrenal which goes on to form oestrone and oestradiol
5. Oestrogens further stimulate the production of arachidonic acid
6. PGs are produced in decidua and fetal membranes
7. Labour is initiated

**NORMAL LABOUR**

Normal labour is characterised by
(i) Regular uterine contractions
(ii) Dilatation of the cervix
(iii) Descent of the presenting part
It encompasses the time from the onset of regular contractions to spontaneous vaginal delivery of the infant (within 24 hours).

**Uterine contractions**
Contractions begin in two 'pace-makers' near the uterotubal junctions. Only one is operative in each contraction which spreads like a wave over the whole uterus. Relaxation begins simultaneously in all areas of the uterus. Labour is characterised by:
(i) Strong and sustained action of the muscle of the uterine fundus
(ii) Less strong contractions of the mid-zone
(iii) Relative inactivity of the lower segment
This fundal dominance increases as labour progresses.

## Cervical dilatation

This occurs from above downwards accompanied by effacement (thinning).

It is caused by coordinated contraction and retraction of the upper segment. The forewaters may act as a hydrostatic wedge and dilatation is facilitated by close apposition of the cervix and presenting part.

## Latent and active phases

The latent phase starts from the onset of regular uterine contractions and ends when the cervix is two to three cm dilated and fully effaced.

It occurs because the thinning of the lower segment and cervix take a lot of uterine work before rapid dilatation can begin.

CERVICAL DILATATION TIME CURVE

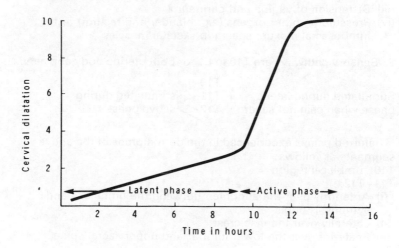

In the active phase the cervix dilates at one to three cm per hour in primigravidae and up to six cm per hour in multigravidae.

Length of first stage of labour.

|  | Mean length in hours Primigravidae | (± 1 SD) Multigravidae |
|---|---|---|
| Latent phase | 9 ± 6 | 5 ± 4 |
| Active phase | 5 ± 3.5 | 2 ± 1.5 |

**Control of uterine activity in labour**
Prostaglandins are likely to be, and oxytocin may be important for
the maintenance of progressive labour. They may be under the
control of the neuro-endocrine 'Ferguson' reflex brought about by
cervical dilatation and vaginal distension.

The autonomic nervous system has little or no motor function.

## PAIN IN LABOUR

Pain is a normal part of labour and delivery although emotional,
cultural and other influences alter individual responses.

*1. Causes*
  (i) Dilatation of the cervix
 (ii) Contraction and distension of the uterus
      Possibly due to the accumulation of pain-producing substances
      during ischaemia
(iii) Distension of vagina and perineum
 (iv) Pressure on other organs (e.g. bladder and rectum) or the
      lumbosacral plexus; spasm in skeletal muscles

2. Sensory pathways are T10 to L1 for both uterine body and cervix

Stimulated during latent    )  T10
phase when pain not severe  )  T11  stimulated during
                               T12  active phase
                               L1

  Referred pain is experienced in the dermatomes of the above
segments as follows:
T10: umbilical region
T11–T12:
  (i) Anteriorly over the abdomen between the umbilicus and
      symphysis pubis
 (ii) Laterally over the iliac crest
(iii) Posterior over the lower lumbar and upper sacral spine.
T12–L1:
  (i) Upper thigh
 (ii) Gluteal region
(iii) Mid-sacral area

*3. Factors affecting pain in childbirth*
*Physical factors* including
  (i) Intensity and duration of contractions
 (ii) Speed of dilatation of cervix
(iii) Vaginal and perineal distension
 (iv) Other factors e.g. age, parity, size of infant, condition of patient

*Physiological factors*
  (i) Pain blocking e.g. customs, culture, preparation, distractive activity
  (ii) Pain aggravating e.g. customs, culture, fear, apprehension, anxiety, ignorance, misinformation
  (iii) Antenatal preparation of the mother and father are very important
(The common midwifery practice of massaging the skin of the lower back or abdomen does modulate pain perception.)

FURTHER READING

Hytten, F. E. & Chamberlain, C. V. P. (1980) *Clinical Physiology in Obstetrics*. Oxford: Blackwell
Bonica J. J. (1975) The nature of pain of parturition. In: Obstetric analgesia-anaesthesia. *Clinics in Obstetrics and Gynaecology*, **2**, 499

## THE TRANSITION FROM FETUS TO NEONATE

Half of the adaptive changes occur within minutes of birth and the rate of adaptation thereafter is slower over the next few days.
  The most immediate demand on the newborn is for oxygen which it can now only obtain by respiration. It has been preparing for this for many weeks in two ways in particular:

1. *Chest wall movements* (fetal breathing)
   These can be detected by ultrasound (and sometimes perceived by the mother). They occur in episodes but the fetus breathes for about 70 per cent of the time at a frequency of 30 to 70 movements per minute

2. *Lung maturation*
   Apart from the development of lung architecture, the most important part of maturation is the production of *surfactant* in the last weeks of pregnancy
   (i) Surfactant is a complex lipoprotein rich in highly saturated lecithins such as dipalmitoyl lecithin
   (ii) It is produced in type II pneumocytes stimulated by cortisol and secreted onto alveolar surfaces

   *Functions of surfactant*
   (i) Maintenance of alveolar stability
   (ii) Reduction of pressure required for initial distension of the lung.

3. *The onset of respiration*
   Among the stimuli producing the first breath are:
   (i) Acute hypoxia due to cessation of maternal oxygen supply
   (ii) The afferent stimuli coming from the outside world

  (iii) Carotid sinus stimulation
The infant's respiratory efforts have two main effects:
  (i) Opening of the pulmonary alveoli
  (ii) Diversion of blood into the pulmonary vascular tree away
       from the foramen ovale and ductus arteriosus.

*4. Circulatory changes at birth*
(a) *Immediate*
        (i) Blood flow ceases in umbilical vessels therefore pressure
            in the ductus venosus drops to zero and right atrial
            pressure falls
       (ii) The raised oxygen tension in the blood produced by
            pulmonary ventilation not only relaxes the smooth
            muscles of the pulmonary arteries (promoting perfusion)
            but also contracts the smooth muscle in the ductus
            arteriosus which closes
      (iii) Increased pulmonary flow increases left atrial pressure
       (iv) The increase in LA pressure and reduction in RA pressure
            apposes the septum primum 'flap' and the septum
            secundum. This closes the foramen ovale
        (v) Adult circulation is established

(b) *Gradual changes*
       (vi) The ductus venosus fibroses forming the *ligamentum
            teres* in the falciform ligament and the *ligamentum
            venosum* connecting the portal vein to the inferior vena
            cava
      (vii) The ductus arteriosus also fibroses to form the
            *ligamentum arteriosum* between the left pulmonary artery
            and aortic arch
     (viii) Fibrinous adhesions between the septa primum and
            secundum become organized and bond permanently

# The puerperium

The puerperium is the period of time over which the whole body, and the genital tract in particular, returns to normal after childbirth. Traditionally it is said to last for six weeks.

The three main features are:
(i) Lactation
(ii) Lochia
(iii) Uterine involution

## LACTATION

1. During pregnancy lactation is prevented by the effect of oestrogen on the breast despite high prolaction levels (see p. 31). Only non-milk colostrum (desquamated epithelium and transudate) is produced
2. *Milk production after delivery*
    (i) The drop in oestrogen allows prolactin to act. Prolactin levels are increased by suckling but only for the first four months of lactation
    (ii) Prolactin maintains protein, casein, fatty acid and lactose content of milk as well as its volume
    (iii) The quantity and quality of milk are also dependent on the action of thyroid hormone, insulin, cortisol, nutrition, and fluid intake
    (iv) Milk is secreted into the alveolar lumen. Breasts begin to fill on the third or fourth postpartum day
    (v) Suckling also suppresses the prolactin inhibitory factor, dopamine, in the hypothalamus

3. *Milk ejection ('let-down')*
    (i) Suckling stimulates an afferent sensory neural arc which causes the paraventricular and supraoptic nuclei of the hypothalamus to synthesise oxytocin then transport it to and release it from the posterior pituitary
    (ii) Oxytocin contracts the myoepithelial cells to empty the alveoli into the ducts and then the areola
    (iii) Frequent emptying maintains production

(iv) Lactation increases the daily energy requirements of the mother from 10.0 megajoules (2400 cal) to 11.5 megajoules (2750 cal)

4. *Cessation of lactation*
   (i) Lack of suckling prevents milk 'let-down' and allows the production of dopamine
   (ii) The swelling due to the milk in the alveoli itself suppresses further production
   (iii) The swollen breast diminishes in size over a few days

5. *Breast feeding*
   (i) The baby can be put to each breast shortly after or within a few hours of birth
   (ii) A small but increasing amount of colostrum will be obtained for the first 36 to 48 hours
   (iii) Suckling stimulates subsequent milk production
   (iv) By day 3 the feeding will be either on demand or 3 to 4 hourly
   (v) The natural demand cycle is usually about 4 hourly
   (vi) The average amount of milk ingested by a normal full-term infant is 20 ml/kg body weight
   (vii) Birthweight is usually regained by day 7 to 10 and about 30 kg/day are added for the next 100 days
   (viii) Breastfeeding is to be encouraged because
       a. It promotes bonding between mother and baby
       b. The fat and protein in breast milk are more readily digested and absorbed than those in cow's milk
       c. Colostrum and breast milk contain antibodies which provide the infant with passive immunity to many infections
       d. Gastroenteritis is rare among breast-fed babies
       e. Milk allergies are avoided
       f. It is safe, cheap and simple
       g. Overfeeding is virtually impossible
       h. The risk of hypocalcaemia with convulsions is reduced
       i. Uterine involution is promoted
       j. The incidence of subsequent breast cancer is reduced
   (ix) The suckling stimulus releases prolactin (see p. 31) which inhibits ovulation. The duration and frequency of suckling are the primary factors in determining when ovulation returns after delivery. Lactation is therefore an important natural method of contraception

## LOCHIA AND UTERINE INVOLUTION

(i) The lochia are mainly blood for the first few days after delivery
(ii) For the next 7 to 10 days they are sero-sanguinous
(iii) Thus remain clear thereafter for up to six weeks
(iv) The total weight of the uterus is reduced by half within seven days of delivery. The mechanism is not sure but the withdrawal of trophic placental hormones and the action of PGs are probably involved

## PSYCHOLOGICAL CHANGES

(i) Postpartum 'blues' can be recognised in at least half of all women delivered
(ii) They tend to develop around the third postpartum day and may last for a few hours or days
(iii) The disturbance is mild characterised by weeping, irritability, variation in mood, a feeling of helplessness, sensitivity to criticism and poor sleep
(iv) Treatment is by support and reassurance rather than medication

FURTHER READING

Beard, R. W., Nathanielsz, (eds.) (1976) *Fetal Physiology and Medicine.* London: W. B. Saunders.
Hytten, F. & Chamberlain, G. (1980) *Clinical Physiology in Obstetrics.* Oxford: Blackwells.

# General clinical physiology

## REACTION TO TRAUMA, HAEMORRHAGE AND SHOCK

The whole body tries to adapt and the changes are mediated by increased activity of the pituitary and adrenal glands.

### Haemorrhage
The effects depend on the amount of blood lost and the speed with which it is lost.

*Phase 1. Early changes*
  *Immediate syncope* may occur as a vasovagal effect. The signs are: hypotension, bradycardia; pallor, cold extremities.

*Redistribution of blood to vital centres*
  (i)   Venous return to the heart and cardiac output fall
  (ii)  Peripheral resistance increases to maintain or restore B.P.
  (iii) Venous reservoir contracts (60 per cent of blood volume is in veins and venules)
  (iv)  Selective arteriolar constriction occurs
        Blood to essential organs is maintained
        Flow to (e.g.) skin, intestines, kidney, spleen and liver fall.
        This occurs by action of the autonomic nervous system, catecholamines and the renin-angiotensin system
  (v)   Acidosis leads to tachypnoea

*Phase 2 — Restoration of blood volume*

*Phase 3 — Replacement of cellular element of blood*

### Shock
Shock is a state of circulatory failure causing impaired tissue perfusion and possible hypoxic damage. In practice it describes a clinical appearance rather than a physiological entity.
The main causes are
  (i)   Fainting (neurogenic)
  (ii)  Low circulating volume (hypovolaemic)
  (iii) 'Pump failure' (cardiogenic)

(iv) Sepsis (bacteraemic)
(v) Adrenocortical insufficiency

## Metabolic response to trauma

**1. Conservation of water and sodium**
(i) Excess secretion of arginine-vasopressin (AVP) causes obligatory oliguria for 48 hours
(ii) Aldosterone causes conservation for several days (depending on the severity of the trauma)

**2. Tissue catabolism**
(i) There is breakdown of depot fat and muscle protein to make materials for wound repair readily available
(ii) Up to 25 G of Nitrogen is lost initially and this cannot be prevented by increased protein intake but is modified by carbohydrate. (This phase can last for up to 10 days if trauma is severe)
(iii) As the protein is broken down potassium is released and hyperkalaemia may occur

**3. Anabolic phase**
As convalescence proceeds nitrogen is retained which allows the body to regain its previous muscle mass.

### Mechanisms
(i) Adrenal corticosteroids rise due to increased ACTH secretion
(ii) In the absence of cortisol the usual metabolic response does not take place
(iii) The normal suppression of ACTH by cortisol is in abeyance
(iv) Adrenaline and noradrenaline are involved in ACTH release and also sensitise the tissues to the action of cortisol
(v) Aldosterone and AVP are involved in the changes in water and sodium

## WOUND HEALING

Wound healing is achieved by:
1. *Repair* in which connective tissue cells migrate and proliferate and form a 'scar'
2. *Regeneration* by which specialised cells re-establish their anatomical integrity and function. Some cells cannot regenerate e.g. nervous system and cardiac muscle
Two types of wound must be considered
1. An incised wound, with little space between the margins which heal by 'primary intention'
2. An open or excised wound which heals by 'secondary' intention

The processes are basically the same: only the timetable is different.

## Programme of wound healing
  (i) Tissue damage and bleeding
 (ii) Clot and 'scab' formation
(iii) Acute inflammatory reaction
(iv) Proliferation and migration of fibroblasts and capillary endothelial cells
 (v) Collagen deposition
(vi) Collagen cross-linkage causing contraction of the wound and scar formation

## Factors which interfere with wound healing
  (i) Poor blood supply
 (ii) Poor apposition of margins
(iii) Infection
(iv) Tumour
 (v) Irradiation
(vi) Protein lack
(vii) Vitamin C deficiency
(viii) Steroids

## FURTHER READING

Ledingham, I. M., Mackay, M. (1978) *Jamieson & Kay's Textbook of Surgical Physiology*, 3rd edn. Edinburgh: Churchill Livingstone

# Index